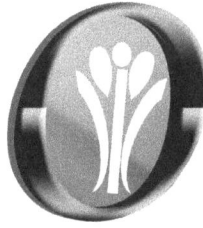

Live Younger
In 8 Simple Steps

By Dr. Eudene Harry

www. LivingHealthyLookingYounger.com

This book is a work of advice and opinion. Neither the author nor the publisher is responsible for actions based on the content of this book. It is not the purpose of this book to include all information about a healthy wellness program. The book should be used as a general health guide and does not replace the care and treatment by a licensed medical professional.

In addition, information and research are continuously changing so please understand what is printed here may not be the most current information available.

Table of Contents

ACKNOWLEDGEMENTS

I would like to thank all the people in my life that played a pivotal role not only in the writing of this book but also to making me the person I am today. To my mother, Celia Francis, thank you for being not only one of my strongest supporters but also my inspiration as well. To my uncle, Ric Francis, I was able to complete medical school due to your generosity of spirit. To my younger brothers, Tyson and Adrian, thank you for always being willing to share your wisdom when I needed it.

I would like to acknowledge my husband for being the driving force in helping to bring this book out of my head onto the pages. He is definitely the wind beneath my wings. To my children, Donovan and Alexis, thank you for teaching me about balance and being in the moment. A special thank you to Dr. Donna Hamilton for being a source of support, inspiration and information from the first day we met in medical school. She is one of the most gifted people with words that I have had the good fortune to call friend.

There are so many other people that played an important role in helping me to get this book published. To Carol Francis, one of the most gifted, creative and artistic individuals I know, thank for being so generous with your time and talent. Katherine Johnson and Lauressa Nelson, your contribution towards the editing process is well noted.

To achieve a balanced life, we all need a support system, a port in the storm, a place to regroup. I wouldn't be where I am today without my good friends and family.

THANK YOU ALL!!!

Introduction

You have heard the old adage: "age is only a number." Imagine for a moment that I have a magic wand and when I wave it in front of you, your body is instantly transformed. Your face looks younger again. The wrinkles, sags and droopy spots in your face disappear. You have a firmer body that looks years younger.

Moreover, your "transformation" is not just skin deep. Your heart and lungs are youthful, your joints are lithe, your muscles are strong and firm, and your immune system is balanced and healthy. Imagine how great you feel. Imagine the strength, the flexibility and the endless supply of energy. You feel like a kid again.

Now let's get back to reality. I don't have a magic wand, but I do have the next best thing – eight simple steps, derived from the science of aging and healthy living, that you can follow to remain as youthful as possible. With these steps, you have the potential to:

- ❖ Melt away body fat and regain a lean appearance
- ❖ Put elasticity back into your skin to minimize wrinkles and regain a youthful glow
- ❖ Grow healthier, stronger, glistening hair and nails
- ❖ Increase your energy levels
- ❖ Improve your memory
- ❖ Increase sexual energy and stamina
- ❖ Develop a stronger immune system

- ❖ Lower your cholesterol levels

- ❖ Build strong and healthy bones

- ❖ Feel the optimism of youth every day

Most people live a life that predisposes them to early aging. This can be turned around without magic potions or pills. Much of what we think of aging, like the lack of energy, frequent illnesses, weight gain, memory loss; the wrinkles in the skin can be the result of a poor diet (high in processed foods and deficient in vitamins, minerals and other micro-nutrients), a lack of exercise, poor skin care, and excessive stress. Did you know that a lack of sleep could make you more prone to being overweight? Did you know that regular exercise could help keep your cognitive skills sharp as a tack? The life you lead and the decisions you make every day are directly responsible for how your body feels and ages.

By making a concerted effort to exercise daily, eat foods that promote longevity, get enough sleep, support the body with the right nutrients, and develop a healthy skin care regime, you can look and feel fabulous, no matter how many birthdays come and go. The goal of this book is to help you lead your healthiest life. Let me show you how by giving you the tools to manage your physical and mental health. Are you ready to get started?

---Dr. Eudene Harry

Simple STEP 1
The Assessment

Kate, a 45-year-old top executive in a Fortune 500 company, walked into my office, looking frazzled and worn. She plopped down in the chair across from me. "I am so tired" were the first words out of her mouth. She went on to tell me that she had everything that most people dreamed of—a great job, two children, a loving husband, and a beautiful home–yet she was unable to enjoy it. She felt she was struggling to get through the day, despite consuming at least five cups of coffee or diet soda. She felt as if she was thinking, seeing and moving through life in a thick fog. Her muscles ached, and her motivation and libido were at an all-time low, with no sign of improvement.

As I delved further into her lifestyle, I learned that Kate ate "on the run," did not exercise, and spent very little time performing self-care. She stayed up late finishing work projects and helping her children with homework, sleeping just five hours a night. Her menstrual cycles were becoming irregular. She gained 20 pounds in one year. Chocolate chip cookies were her stress management tools. She was diagnosed with high blood pressure and taking medication. Kate's family history included osteoporosis, heart disease and diabetes. With good reason, she expressed concern about developing these diseases, as she got older.

Although her life looked great from the outside, Kate felt like she was falling apart on the inside. "I want my life back," she said. "When I look in the mirror, I don't recognize the person looking back at me. If one more person tells me I look tired, I am going to scream," she lamented.

The dark shadows under Kate's eyes and her dull, lackluster skin were evidence of her extreme exhaustion and tension. Her unintentional, habitual frowning made the lines between her eyebrows more pronounced, giving the impression of anger or sadness. She was also experiencing a mild loss of elasticity in the face, producing a sagging, downturned appearance.

During her examination, Kate's blood pressure was 150/93, her resting pulse rate 85 beats per minute, and her breathing pattern appeared very shallow. At 5 feet 4 inches and weighing 160 pounds, her body mass index (BMI) was 27.5, indicating that she was overweight. Her waist circumference of 35 inches was large for her frame, and her body fat percentage measured 34.

Kate was in need of a healthy start – both physically and mentally. Together we created a detailed, structured plan to rehabilitate her mind, body and spirit.

Many people think aging is all about loss. I like to think that aging is all about change. With change, one thing leaves to make room for another–aging offers us the opportunity to trade years for wisdom. We all age–that is a given–but aging can be about living longer in a healthier way. Take the right actions today, and you will be able to retain your health and vitality, age gracefully, and live a long, happy life.

Many of the strategies in this book focus on identifying possible causes of accelerated aging, giving you easy steps to reduce the signs of aging, and slowing down the process by repairing damage from free radicals by modifying your risk factors. A sedentary lifestyle, poor diet and stress can all contribute to chronic diseases.

The first step in evaluating your body's physical and mental condition is to schedule a full assessment with your physician. A visit to your doctor is an opportunity not only to learn about your health, but also to get a better understanding of your risk for developing future diseases. Your doctor will order a series of tests collectively referred as an annual screening evaluation. These tests evaluate liver function, kidney function, cholesterol levels, and blood sugar levels. They also check for anemia and white cell abnormalities (immune system) and may include a thyroid screening. Often these tests can help identify whether or not a disease is already present. Physicians who focus on wellness and youthful aging will further evaluate patterns of nutrient deficiencies, hormonal imbalances, and inflammatory markers that could indicate increased risk of chronic illnesses, such as cardiovascular disease, stroke and diabetes.

Medical and nutritional sciences have done some amazing work identifying markers to help physicians get ahead of chronic illness. In this chapter, I explore some recently identified markers and how they help a wellness physician customize a personalized anti-aging plan for a patient.

First, let's look at some of the individual risk factors.

HEART DISEASE

Heart disease is one of the leading causes of death in men and women. According to the Centers for Disease Control (CDC), more than one million people suffer heart attacks every year. In 2010, it was estimated that heart disease cost an estimated $316 billion in health care costs. Heart disease is expensive both physically and financially.

Many factors contribute to the development of coronary artery disease, which ultimately leads to a heart attack or stroke. While there is no single difference between people who develop heart disease and those who don't, evaluating and addressing known risk factors is prudent to reducing risk.

Recent studies suggest that inflammation plays a major role in this process, but what triggers the inflammation may vary. Some studies point to bacterial and viral culprits. In addition, certain foods, elevated cholesterol levels, and other lifestyle factors, like smoking, have been implicated as factors. Short-lived inflammation is the body's way of fighting viruses, wounds, bacteria, chemical irritants, and other types of trauma. After injury or damage to a tissue within the body, immune cells rush in, and release compounds to destroy the culprit that causing the damage or infection. When the condition is healed, the immune system response usually goes away, but sometimes inflammation can persist.

Inflammation is not the only risk factor for disease. Other common risk factors that physicians will evaluate during an assessment include:

*Fibrinogen levels: A blood-clotting protein known as fibrinogen has been shown to play a role in the development of heart disease. Fibrinogen plays an important role to help blood to clot. In healthy adults, fibrinogen prevents excessive bleeding if we get a cut or wound. However, elevated fibrinogen levels may increase the formation of clots in blood vessels, and increase the risk of heart attacks and strokes. A Scottish study cited in *Journal of Epidemiology* (1993) showed a strong correlation between elevated fibrinogen levels and heart disease. This correlation appears to be higher in men than women.

*Infectious Bacteria:** There are two main bacteria associated with the formation of arterial plaque. They are called Helicobacter pylori and Chlamydia pneumoniae. The presence of the bacteria Helicobacter pylori (H. pylori) is normally associated with ulcers, but has also been found in the arterial plaque buildup in a significant number of heart attack patients. If you have elevated CRP, your wellness physician may check for the presence of H. Pylori bacteria.

Chlamydia pneumoniae is another bacterium that may be implicated in heart disease. It is responsible for nearly 10 percent of pneumonia cases. This bacterium can result in chronic low-level inflammation in the blood vessels that can make the heart vessels more vulnerable to developing fatty deposits and plaque formation.

Family history: Family history is considered a significant risk factor for heart disease. One study published in *Journal of Epidemiology* in 2001 noted that women with a family history of heart disease were three times more likely to develop the disease than those without a family history. Having a brother or sister with heart disease is associated with a higher risk than having one parent with heart disease. Another important discovery, as reported in the *European Heart Journal* and the *British Heart Journal*, implicates age and risk. Risk factors increase depending on the age of the relative and how many family members are affected. It is important to consider the environmental components to family history, keeping in mind that many families tend to grow up with similar eating, activity and lifestyle patterns, which can impact other risk factors, such as cholesterol, and increase the risk of heart disease.

*Smoking and drug abuse: It is estimated that as much as 30 percent of heart disease in the U.S. is attributed to cigarette smoking, according to the U.S. Department of Health and Human Services. Smoking also increases the risk of stroke, peripheral vascular disease, lung disease, osteopenia, and many other chronic illnesses. The good news is that it takes a relatively short amount of time to experience some benefits of smoking cessation. For example, there is a 50 percent reduction in risk of another heart attack for those that stop smoking after their first heart attack, as reported in a study published in the *British Heart Journal*. Looks like the old adage, "it's never too late to change" applies when it comes to smoking.

Illicit drug use is quickly becoming a significant risk factor for heart attacks. Certain drugs, such as cocaine, that act as stimulants on the cardiovascular system can also precipitate heart attacks without any significant blockage to the artery.

*Activity Level: The American Heart Association states that a sedentary lifestyle is one of the major risk factors contributing to the development of heart disease. This is why I am a firm believer in the benefits of daily exercise to maintain a healthy weight. Many studies show that there are significant health concerns associated with obesity including heart disease, hypertension, diabetes, and certain types of cancers. Exercise may have a direct impact on maintaining healthy blood pressure levels by inducing production of a substance called nitric oxide. This substance helps to induce vascular smooth cell relaxation that can contribute to lower blood pressure values. We will review the many benefits of simply getting up and moving in Chapter 4.

*Diabetes: Diabetes remains an independent risk factor for cardiovascular disease. Patients with diabetes typically face a worst-case prognosis when a cardiovascular event occurs.

This means that if you suffer a heart attack and you are a diabetic, your chances of a full recovery diminish significantly. We'll explore diabetes as a risk factor in further detail later in this chapter.

After evaluating all of your risk factors for heart disease, your doctor may decide to perform additional tests to further evaluate the health of your cardiovascular system. The initial screening for the heart is called the electrocardiogram (EKG or ECG). If ECG results or medical history indicates, further evaluation can include a stress test, echocardiogram (ultrasound of the heart) or cardiac computed tomography (CT) heart scans. A CT scan is an imaging test that produces cross-sectional views of the heart's anatomy, coronary circulation, and major vessels by combining multiple X-ray images. When a patient is diagnosed with heart disease, one type of CT scan a physician may order is called the calcium-score screening heart scan. It notes calcium deposits found in atherosclerotic plaque in the coronary arteries: the higher the calcium scores in asymptomatic individuals, the higher the future chances of developing heart disease. While it is a helpful diagnostic tool, concerns have been raised about its costs and the exposure patients receive to ionizing radiation during the X-ray evaluation, which may possibly contribute to DNA damage and an increased risk of cancer. Physicians and patients should always assess the risk-to-benefit ratio before performing this study.

Your physician may order other key laboratory tests to help assess your risk for heart disease. These include:

1. **High Sensitivity C-Reactive Protein (hs-CRP)**
Hs-CRP is a marker for inflammation that is specific to the blood vessels. The Physicians Health Study (PHS) and Harvard Women's Health Study (HWHS) note an association

between elevated hs-CRP results and heart disease. The PHS found that elevated hs-CRP results were associated with a threefold increase in the risk of a heart attack. The HWHS found that the hs-CRP test was more accurate than cholesterol levels in assessing the risk of heart disease among women.

While the test can pinpoint heart disease, it is not able to identify the source of inflammation. Hidden infections, such as Helicobacter pylori (H. pylori) and even low-grade or undetected dental infections can contribute to elevated levels of this inflammatory marker.

Overweight patients tend to have higher hs-CRP values. Fat has been shown to increase the production of inflammatory hormones. A study published in *Diabetes Care*, May 2003, found a strong association between increased levels of hemoglobin A1c (HbA1c) test—a marker tracking control of diabetes—and the hs-CRP test. This suggests that the inflammatory response associated with diabetes mellitus may also play in a role increasing cardiac risk factors. If a patient's hs-CRP numbers are elevated, a physician may decide that further studies are needed to identify the source of the inflammation.

According to the American Heart Association and the CDC, patients with hs-CRP levels less than 1.0 mg/L are deemed low risk for heart disease. Those exhibiting levels of 1.0 to 3.0 mg/L are at average risk, and individuals with levels above 3.0 mg/L are at high risk. In wellness medicine, we strive to reduce risk as much as possible. If levels are significantly elevated, then specific causes—such as autoimmune diseases, certain forms of arthritis and infections—may need to be investigated.

2. Homocysteine levels:

Homocysteine is an amino acid formed when another amino acid called methionine is metabolized. Methionine cannot be made in the body and must be obtained through the diet, making it an essential amino acid. Methionine can help neutralize free radicals that damage healthy cells and tissues and lead to organ and structural damage.

Methionine can also convert cysteine, an important amino acid in the formation of glutathione, the body's powerhouse detoxifier. Homocysteine is an intermediary step in this process. Inadequate amounts of folic acid or vitamins B6 or B12 can slow the formation of methionine, causing elevated homocysteine levels. Too much homocysteine can be toxic to the vascular system and is associated with atherosclerosis, according to a 2001 study in the *European Heart Journal* (v. 22, 77-71).

Lipid Panel

High levels of blood fats known as lipoproteins and triglycerides are associated with an increased risk of heart disease. Lipoproteins are molecules that transport cholesterol in the bloodstream. There are many types, but the two most common are low-density lipoproteins (LDL), known as bad cholesterol, and high-density lipoproteins (HDL), known as good cholesterol. High levels of LDL can lead to the formation of fatty plaques that can narrow the arteries and reduce blood flow, and contribute to atherosclerosis.

By carrying cholesterol away from the arteries and back to the liver for processing, HDL is thought to protect the body against vascular disease. However, a sedentary lifestyle, poor nutrition, and in some cases, genetics, can have a negative impact on healthy levels. Recently researchers discovered that there are several types of LDL and HDL molecules. Certain subgroups of HDL are thought to offer more protection against heart disease than others. The same is true for LDL; some forms seem to be more damaging to blood vessels.

The Vertical Auto Profile-II (VAP-II) cholesterol test offers significant advantages over the standard cholesterol testing. This test tells physicians exactly how much LDL is present in the blood stream. This is important because routine cholesterol testing gives an estimated or calculated value of the bad cholesterol. If fats in the blood are too high, then the value of the LDL measured in a regular cholesterol test can be inaccurate. To improve the accuracy of the regular cholesterol test it must performed after fasting. Because the VAP test directly measures LDL cholesterol, it will deliver accurate results even if you are not fasting.

Studies also suggest that the size of the particle is also important. The smaller the LDL particle, the more it contributes to plaque formation and heart disease. In the case of HDL, or "good cholesterol," smaller particles may not be as protective as larger ones. The VAP-II test is able to provide additional information on the size of the LDL and HDL particles and allow physicians to better assess risk for coronary artery disease.

A lipid panel also measures triglycerides, or lipids (fats) that bind to proteins to form the high and low-density lipoproteins. As with LDL, high triglyceride levels are associated with atherosclerosis and heart disease. Eating too many fatty foods, drinking too much alcohol, or having high insulin levels can result in high triglyceride levels.

DIABETES

As mentioned earlier, diabetes is a key risk factor that physicians look for during an assessment. Diabetes mellitus, or diabetes, is the name for a group of diseases characterized by high blood glucose levels that result when the body is unable to produce and/or use insulin. There are two types, commonly referred to as Type 1 and Type 2.

In Type 1 diabetes, the insulin-producing cells in the pancreas are destroyed by the patient's own immune system and the body does not produce insulin. Insulin is a hormone that is needed to convert sugar, starches and other food into energy needed to sustain daily life. Insulin controls the amount of sugar (glucose) in the blood and the rate glucose is absorbed into the cells. If insulin production goes down, then blood sugar levels can rise, sometimes to dangerous levels. For many Type 1 diabetics, insulin replacement is necessary. Type 1 diabetes, once known as juvenile diabetes, is often diagnosed in children and young adults. Only five percent of people with diabetes have this form of the disease.

Type 2 diabetes is the most common form and is one of the fastest growing health threats in the U.S. today. It not only threatens adults, but children as well. **The statistics are grim: every 20 seconds, someone in the U.S. is diagnosed with Type 2 diabetes.** Millions of Americans have been diagnosed, and millions more don't even realize that they are at high risk. Type 2 diabetes is most common among African Americans, Latinos, Native Americans, Asian Americans, Native Hawaiians and Pacific Islanders, as well as the elderly and obese population.

With Type 2 diabetes, either the body does not produce enough insulin or the cells do not respond to the insulin. Type 2 diabetes often begins with higher than normal insulin levels. It is believed that this form of diabetes is a result of poor diet and lifestyle choices. When we consume a diet high in refined carbohydrates and simple sugars, it prompts our bodies to overproduce and release too much insulin. Insulin acts as a "key" to open the door and allows glucose (sugar) to enter cells to be converted to fuel needed to power our bodies. The more sugars and refined carbohydrates we consume, the higher our blood sugar and insulin levels.

Abnormal Insulin Responses

In some people, this increase in insulin may cause a significant drop in blood sugar levels that can result in hypoglycemia. When someone becomes hypoglycemic, they may exhibit symptoms such as feeling shaky, clammy, sweaty, and anxious. They may also experience heart palpitations, and their ability to reason can become impaired. This may occur in part because low blood sugar levels may trigger a panic response in the body causing it to release high levels of adrenaline. Adrenaline then causes the additional symptoms in the body.

Over time, if the cells are continually exposed to high levels of insulin, they may become resistant, and require the production of additional insulin to remove excess sugars from the blood. This occurs because the cells that have been exposed to excessive levels of the hormone compensate by decreasing the number of receptors (doors) available to accept it. That means insulin becomes less efficient at opening the "doors" to allow glucose into the cells, causing the pancreas to produce additional insulin in an effort to compensate.

Eventually this process fails and blood sugar levels begin to rise, and the body's cells cannot produce as much energy. Excess sugars floating in the blood attaches to protein structures in tissues and cell membranes, causing damage by changing the structure and the function of these tissues and cells. A good illustration of this process is similar to what happens when you heat egg whites (protein). When the egg white is cooked, the structure changes so that it is no longer fluid and moveable. While this may be a good thing before eating an egg, it is detrimental to the proteins in the living body because their function often depends upon the maintenance of the original structure and fluidity.

If blood sugar levels are too high, it is known as hyperglycemia. Persistently elevated blood sugar levels can lead to the diagnoses of diabetes. If it is not properly controlled, diabetes can lead to heart disease, kidney disease, nerve damage, changes in vision or blindness, infections, and delayed healing of injuries. Excessive levels of insulin and high blood sugars cause damage to the body.

In order to evaluate the risk of developing Type 2 diabetes, physicians will perform several lab work and studies. These include:

1. Glucose levels (preferably fasting)

Fasting blood sugar levels should be measured within 6 to 8 hours after eating. The measurement is milligrams of glucose per 1/10 liter (mg/dl) of blood.

- 70 to 100 is considered normal
- 100 to 125 indicates impaired glucose tolerance/borderline diabetes
- 126 and over for two to three days suggests diabetes

2. HbA1c Levels

The hemoglobin A1c (HbA1c) test measures the glycosylated hemoglobin in the blood, the substance in red blood cells formed when glucose attaches to hemoglobin. Since red blood cells live for approximately three months, this test estimates the level of a patient's blood sugar levels (glucose) over the previous three-month period. The higher your blood sugar levels, the higher HbA1c. A normal level is less than 5.6 percent. Any level above 5.6 may be reason for concern and should be corrected, even though HbA1c above 6.5 percent is the official threshold to diagnose diabetes. If you have diabetes, you should try to keep your HbA1c level at or below 7 percent.

3. Fasting Insulin Levels

This refers to a patient's insulin level after fasting for at least eight hours. The normal range varies by laboratory performing test, but 5-20 mcU/ml during fasting (mcU/ml refers to micro unit per millimeter) is preferred. However, many wellness physicians believe that a level higher than 10 is indicative of insulin resistance. Remember: the idea is prevention of the disease, not reaction to the disease.

4. Glucose Tolerance Test with Insulin

This oral glucose tolerance test (OGTT) is often performed to screen expectant mothers between 24 and 28 weeks of pregnancy for gestational diabetes. There are significant health risks to both mom and baby if hyperglycemia or diabetes is not diagnosed quickly. The test is more sensitive in identifying patients with glucose control issues, and may be used in cases where diabetes is suspected, despite a normal fasting blood glucose level. As diabetes cases continue to rise, this test is a very cost-effective tool to prevent and diagnose patients.

5. Adinopectin Levels

Adiponectin is a protein hormone produced by the adipocytes (fat cells) and involved with metabolic processes such as glucose regulation and fatty acid catabolism. A study in the July 2009 *Journal of Pediatrics* found that adinopectin levels are lower in obese insulin-resistant individuals, suggesting that insulin sensitivity (i.e., the way the cells use insulin to take in glucose) is improved by adiponectin and it may offer anti-inflammatory benefits. A patient's adiponectin level has been added to the list of markers that may help determine who is at risk for insulin resistance and Type 2 diabetes.

The Mediterranean diet has been shown to increase the level of this hormone, while a carbohydrate-rich diet decreases it, according to reports in the *Journal of Nutritional Biochemistry* (April 2010) and the *Journal of Clinical Investigation*. This test along with HbA1c, insulin and glucose levels may help your physician determine your future risk of developing Type 2 diabetes.

Metabolic Syndrome

Metabolic syndrome is defined as a cluster of conditions that include increased blood pressure, elevated insulin levels, excess body fat around the waist, and abnormal cholesterol levels. When these symptoms occur simultaneously, they increase your risk for heart disease, stroke and diabetes.

Having metabolic syndrome means you have three or more disorders related to your metabolism diagnosed at the same time, including:

• Being **overweight,** particularly around your waist.

- A systolic (top number) **blood pressure** measurement higher than 120 millimeters of mercury (mmHg) or a diastolic (bottom number) measurement higher than 80 mmHg.

- An elevated level of the blood fat called **triglycerides** and a low level of high-density lipoprotein (HDL) or "good cholesterol."

- **Resistance to insulin**, a hormone that helps to regulate the amount of sugar in your body.

OSTEOPOROSIS

The third risk assessment physicians will review is osteoporosis, defined as the thinning of the bone with a reduction in bone mass due to loss of bone tissue. Many factors can affect the rate osteoporosis occurs. A wellness physician can determine your risk of this disease by ordering specific laboratory tests and studies. The physician should obtain detailed social and nutritional history by reviewing factors that can affect a patient's risk for developing osteoporosis. Some risk factors can be modified, while others cannot.

Ok, so now we've completed the evaluation for risk factors. Most of you are probably asking, "What steps can I take right now to change?" Here are some contributing risk factor behaviors and lifestyle modifications you can start today.

- **Boost your calcium intake.** A lifelong lack of calcium can play a major role in the development of osteoporosis. Low calcium intake contributes to diminished bone density, early bone loss, and an increased risk of fractures.

- **Cut out tobacco use**. There's no better time to stop.

Although its exact role in osteoporosis is not clearly understood, tobacco has been shown to contribute to weak bones.

- **Manage eating disorders.** Women and men with anorexia nervosa or bulimia are at a higher risk of developing low bone density due to significant nutrient deficiencies.

- **Get up and move.** People who spend a lot of time sitting have a higher risk of osteoporosis than their more active peers. Weight-bearing exercises are beneficial to maintain strong bones, but walking, running, jumping, dancing and weightlifting are also helpful for building healthy bones.

- **Lower excessive alcohol consumption.** Regular consumption of more than two alcoholic drinks a day increases your risk of osteoporosis. One theory is that alcohol can interfere with the body's ability to absorb calcium.

- **Cut the fizz.** Researchers at Tufts University found that women who consumed three or more regular or diet sodas daily had a four percent decrease in hipbone density.

- **Monitor corticosteroid medications:** Long-term use of corticosteroid medications, such as prednisone, cortisone and dexamethasone can lead to bone loss and osteoporosis. These medications are common treatments for chronic conditions, such as asthma, rheumatoid arthritis and lupus. If you need to take a steroid medication for an extended period, your doctor should monitor your bone density and recommend other drugs to help prevent bone loss.

- **Monitor other medications.** Increased risk of osteoporosis is also associated with certain medications. These include long-term use of aromatase inhibitors to treat breast cancer, the cancer treatment drug methotrexate, some anti-seizure medications, acid-blocking drugs called proton pump inhibitors, and aluminum-containing antacids. The antidepressant medications called selective serotonin reuptake inhibitors (SSRIs) have also been associated with increased risk of osteoporosis, according to studies published in the *Archives of Internal Medicine* (2007).

While there are plenty of changes you can make to your diet and lifestyle now, some factors that can't be modified. These factors include race, gender and chronic medical conditions.

Risk Factors that Cannot Be Changed:

  Being a woman: Fractures from osteoporosis are almost twice as common in women as in men

  Getting older: The older you get, the greater your risk of osteoporosis. A decrease in hormones as we age affects bone health in men and women. Post-menopausal women lose bone mass at an accelerated rate. Hormone replacement therapy has been shown to offset some of these changes.

  Race: The risk of osteoporosis is highest among Caucasians and people of Asian descent.

  Family history: Individuals whose parents or siblings have osteoporosis, especially if they also have a family history of fractures, are at greatest risk.

  Frame size: Men and women who are exceptionally thin

(with a body mass index of 19 or less) or have small body frames tend to have a higher risk because they may have less bone mass as they age.

*__Hyperthyroidism:__ Too much thyroid hormone can cause bone loss, because either the thyroid is overactive (hyperthyroidism) or excessive amounts of thyroid hormone medication have been taken to treat an underactive thyroid (hypothyroidism).

*__Stomach and weight-loss surgery__ can affect your body's ability to absorb calcium.

*__Other Conditions:__ Conditions such as Crohn's disease, celiac disease, hyperparathyroidism (too much parathyroid hormone in the body) and Cushing's disease (a rare disorder where the adrenal glands produce excessive corticosteroid hormones) significantly increase the risk of osteoporosis.

Fractures are the most frequent and serious complication of osteoporosis. They often occur in the spine or hip, bones that directly support the body's weight. Hip fractures can often result from a fall. However, if there is enough bone mass loss, the hip can spontaneously break, causing the individual to fall. Although most people do relatively well with modern surgical treatment, hip fractures can result in disability and even death from postoperative complications, especially in older adults. The mortality after hip fracture remains approximately 25% within 1 year post operatively, despite modern medical intervention. Wrist fractures also are common in these patients. In many patients with osteoporosis, spinal fractures can occur, even without a fall or trauma. The vertebrae can simply become so weakened that they begin to compress or collapse. Compression fractures can cause severe pain and require a long recovery. Multiple compression fractures can lead to a loss in height and an abnormal, convex curvature of the spine that creates a bulge at the upper back. This stooped or hunched posture is known as kyphosis.

Physicians use several tools to evaluate the risk of osteoporosis in patients. Your physician may order one or more of the following studies:

- **Vitamin D :** A deficiency is detected by testing the blood for levels of vitamin D_{25}, also known as cholecalciferol. One study at the University of Toronto suggests that 800IU of Vitamin D daily could reduce hip fractures by 38 percent. If you do not receive enough sun exposure or do not supplement with enough vitamin D_3, then deficiency is likely.
- **Dual energy x-ray absorptiometry (DEXA) scan:** For individuals considered at risk based on history, age (over 50) or laboratory evaluations, a physician will usually order a DEXA scan to evaluate bone density.
- **Deoxypyridinoline Crosslink** (also called D-Pyrilinks or Pyrilinks-D): This test is performed using blood or urine samples and measures a patient's bone resorption rate (how quickly bone is breaking down). It is a valuable tool to measure the effectiveness of treatment, rather than depending solely upon the DEXA scan, which may take one to two years to show improved results.

HORMONE ASSESSMENT

No healthy aging evaluation is complete without assessing a patient's hormonal levels. Hormones play a significant role not only in the way we look and feel, but also our overall health. Balancing our hormone levels can go a long way in optimizing our health.

What are Hormones?

Hormones are substances produced in one part of the body and carried by the blood stream to other parts. They affect physiological change and activity throughout all of the body's individual cells.

There are many different types of hormones produced by the individual organs in the body. Many of us are familiar with thyroid hormones and sex hormones such as estrogen and testosterone as we approach menopause or andropause (yes men, you can suffer the effects of diminishing hormones as well). However, there are many other important hormones in the body to monitor, such as insulin (which helps control blood sugar levels) and cortisol (which plays an important role in our stress response mechanism).

An imbalance in any one of these hormones can have an adverse effect on our health and well being, and can impair the functions of other hormones. As if that is not complicated enough, it turns out that the body's neurotransmitters (chemicals produced by the brain that affect our moods) play an important role in helping hormones function optimally and vice versa. Just one hormone out of balance can present multiple symptoms because of its effect on the other systems in the body.

To get a better understanding of why hormonal balance plays

such an integral part of your optimal health, I will review some common hormones and some signs and symptoms of deficiency and/or excess. We have already discussed insulin and the crucial role it plays in maintaining proper blood sugar balance (glucose). To review, insulin helps blood sugars enter into the cells so it can be converted or stored as energy and is produced by the pancreas. If insulin levels become too high, then a patient's risk for metabolic syndrome, Type 2 diabetes, and heart disease increases.

Thyroid hormones are also play an important role in helping maintain optimal health. These hormones are produced by the thyroid gland, a butterfly shaped organ located in the front of the neck. They are formed from a tyrosine amino acid molecule and iodine molecules. There are two metabolically active forms of thyroid hormones: thyroxine (T4) and triiodothyronine (T3). The numbers donate the number of iodine molecules associated with each of the tyrosine components. The T3 hormone is formed from the T4 hormone, and is estimated to be 3-4 times more metabolically active than the T4 hormone.

Most of the thyroid hormones in the body are bound to a carrier protein. Think of a carrier protein as a bag that gathers and holds hormones. Hormones carried in this bag are not available for the body to use and considered inactive. Hormones not bound to the carrier protein are referred as a free hormone. These hormones affect the metabolic function in the body. It is important to evaluate not only a patient's total amount of thyroid hormones during an assessment, but also the available (free) amount of hormones.

Hypothyroidism (defined as a deficiency of thyroid hormones) is associated with weight gain, hypertension, elevated cholesterol levels, decreased contractility of the heart muscle (which could lead to congestive heart failure), fatigue, depression, myxedema, hair loss, infertility, cold intolerance, and generalized weakness. Hypothyroidism is often the result of a decreased production of thyroid hormones by the thyroid gland. The most common cause of hypothyroidism in the United States today is an autoimmune disorder known as Hashimotos Thyroiditis. This condition allows the body's immune system to attack the thyroid gland and compromises its ability to produce thyroid hormones. Another cause of hypothyroidism is iodine deficiency and is the most common cause of low thyroid function worldwide. The incidence of hypothyroidism increases with age and among females. Hyperthyroidism (defined as a production of excess thyroid hormones) can cause other health issues as well. Patients can experience palpitations, irregular heartbeat, chest pain, anxiety, muscle weakness, heat intolerance, weight loss, and even hair loss.

There are several laboratory tests to evaluate your thyroid. Here are some of the more common studies used by physicians:

*TSH (Thyroid stimulating hormone): This hormone is secreted by one of the master glands in the brain known as the pituitary gland. This hormone then acts on the thyroid gland to induce the formation of thyroid hormones. If there is insufficient hormone production, the brain detects the drop and increases production of the TSH in an attempt to boost hormone production. An elevated TSH level is an indicator of a low thyroid function or hypothyroidism; the same is true for hyperthyroidism. If there is over production of the thyroid hormones, the brain detects this rise and significantly decreases TSH production. Therefore, a low TSH indicates an over production of thyroid hormones.

*Free T4 (thyroxine): This is the most abundant thyroid hormone and often the one that is replaced in the treatment of hypothyroidism.

*Free T3 (triiodothyronine): This form of thyroid hormone is derived from T4 and has three to four times the metabolic activity of T4. Studies suggest that some individuals may benefit from this form of thyroid hormone replacement along with T4.

*TPO/Thyroglobulin antibodies: This process involves screening antibodies to detect if the immune system has formed significant antibodies against thyroid proteins. This could indicate possible autoimmune thyroiditis (inflammation of thyroid).

Keep in mind there may be other causes of hypothyroidism and hyperthyroidism that are beyond the scope of this book. It is recommended that you discuss these with your physician if you have any concerns or questions.

SEX HORMONE ASSESSMENT

The evaluation of sex hormones is much more controversial and complex. Simply stated, sex hormones are hormones that affect the growth and function of reproduction organs. However, sex hormones are anything but simple, and it is not possible to detail all of the hormones in this book. After all, science is still trying to figure out all of the nuances and functions of these powerful chemicals.

As we approach the five years prior and even the five years after menopause begins, women may experience signs and symptoms of hormonal imbalance. Often these go unrecognized as characteristics of a hormonal imbalance.

For example, cholesterol levels may start to increase, and women suffer from insomnia, anxiety or even depression. Studies show that a lack of sleep, depression and elevated cholesterol can lead to not only weight gain, but also an increased risk of Type 2 diabetes and even heart disease. This is just one example of how hormonal imbalances affect overall health and well-being. An evaluation of the sex hormones estrogen, testosterone and progesterone (especially around menopausal years) may help your physician to determine if a hormonal imbalance is contributing to your symptomology.

EVALUATING SEX HORMONES:
There are several laboratory tests available today for physicians to evaluate sex hormones. These include:

*FSH (follicular stimulating hormone)/LH (leutinizing hormone): Like the thyroid, these hormones are secreted by the pituitary gland in the brain. They trigger release of the egg from the ovary and stimulate the egg to produce estrogen and progesterone. Similar to the thyroid there is a feedback mechanism in place and these hormones can be measured. When there is not enough estrogen released, the levels of FSH rise in efforts to try to increase estrogen production from the ovaries. Around menopause, the ovarian release of eggs and production of hormones diminishes significantly and FSH levels rise. A high FSH can be a good indication of low hormone production. FSH and LH are also secreted by the male's pituitary as well. LH helps stimulate the production of testosterone and FSH helps with the process of sperm formation.

*Estrogen: It is considered the primary female sex hormone, but it is also produced in men in lower quantities. Estrogen is primarily produced in the ovaries by the action of an enzyme on the hormone testosterone (yes, you heard correctly – the male hormone). As men get older, there may be an increase in the conversion of testosterone to estrogen, thus lowering testosterone levels and increasing estrogen levels. This shift may exacerbate symptoms such as a low libido and fatigue. Estrogen can also be produced in smaller quantities in other areas of the body, like the liver, adrenal glands, and even in fat cells.

There are actually three types of estrogens: estradiol, estrone and estriol. Estradiol and estrone are considered the most metabolically active forms. Estradiol and estrone can switch back and forth in the body. Estriol cannot be made into the other two hormones and is considered a very weak estrogen. A few studies have suggested that estriol may even offer some protection against estradiol and estrone's ability to make cells grow faster. The process would allow estriol, as a weaker estrogen, to take the place of the stronger estrogens and reduce its ability to fully function. However, some recent studies question whether this hypothesis might be premature.

There is a discovery of a fourth estrogen called E4 (estetrol). This hormone is pregnancy specific and only produced by the fetus's liver around the 20-week gestation period. It seems to have similar properties to the other estrogens. It can support bone density and strength and has estrogenic effects on the uterus and vagina, such as maintaining muscle tone and strength and lubrication. One exciting discovery about this estrogen was reported in a rat model study. It showed that E4 prevented and suppressed mammary tumor growth, similar to the breast cancer drug Tamoxifen. This finding may prove promising for women with hormone sensitive cancers or who are experiencing significant estrogen deficiency symptoms. Estetrol also seems to work well as a contraceptive.

We have discussed some of the signs of estrogen deficiency, but we also need to be aware of the concerns surrounding excess estrogen. Too much estrogen is linked to an increased risk of autoimmune disorders such as SLE (lupus) and an exacerbation of other autoimmune disorders such as rheumatoid arthritis. Excess estrogen can increase risk of endometrial cancer (lining of the uterus) and there is concern about an increased risk of breast cancer. Excessive estrogen can also exacerbate the growth of fibroids and contribute to heavy menstrual cycles. In males, excessive estrogen is linked to decreased sperm production and an increased risk of some forms of prostate cancer.

*Testosterone: It may be regarded as the male hormone, but it is also produced in women. In men, testosterone has been shown to decrease about 1 percent every year after the age of 30. In some men the decrease in testosterone remains asymptomatic. However, low testosterone levels in other men can produce symptoms of depression, low libido, insomnia, fatigue, decreased bone density, weight gain and accelerated muscle loss. Men may even experience significant hot flashes and enlarged breast tissue (remember estrogen levels potentially increases with age as well). In women, testosterone has been shown to increase sexual activity and desire. Excessive testosterone can contribute to symptoms of Polycystic Ovarian Syndrome (PCOS). Signs and symptoms of this disorder include excessive hair growth, weight gain, as well as insulin and blood sugar imbalances. Too much testosterone can also cause acne and oily skin.

*Progesterone: This hormone is primarily considered a female hormone that is produced by the ovaries during ovulation (release of the egg). One of the main functions of progesterone is to prepare the uterine lining for implantation of pregnancy. If pregnancy does not occur, then progesterone levels drop and menstruation occurs.

Studies suggest that progesterone may play an important role in protecting the brain in both female and male patients. A double blind placebo study published in the 2006 *Annals of Emergency Medicine* found progesterone reduced mortality from traumatic brain injuries by 50 percent and significantly improved functionality in those with moderate brain injuries. This finding was reported in both men and women. It was also noted that progesterone was tolerated as well as a placebo and deemed safe. Another study published in *British Medical Journal* also linked post-partum depression to a rapid fall in progesterone levels. These studies suggest that progesterone may play a significantly higher role in brain function than previously reported.

In studies with mice, progesterone was shown to support the formation of the protective fatty layer that covers nerve cells (myelin sheath). It has been noted that symptoms of multiple sclerosis (a disease that destroys the myelin protection that covers nerves) can improve significantly during pregnancy, a time when progesterone levels are high. Studies also show that progesterone may also help with anxiety and protect against uterine cancer. A few studies suggest that it may also decrease the excessive growth of breast cells. Like any hormone in the body, it is possible to take progesterone in excess or be intolerant. For example, some studies suggest that progesterone could possibly exacerbate insulin resistance in some individuals.

While there is a mountain of evidence that indicates low hormones contribute to depression, low libido, anxiety, hair loss, dry skin, vaginal dryness (in women), premature aging of the skin, hot flashes, insomnia, and osteopenia, there is much more controversy surrounding hormone replacement therapy (HRT). Researchers are divided whether HRT is effective, safe and necessary for patients. My opinion is that HRT needs to be made on a case-by-case basis with each patient. Many factors affect hormonal balance. For example, some studies show that moderate to heavy consumption of alcohol actually has an effect on the hormones estradiol and progesterone. It can decrease the levels of progesterone or increase levels of estradiol, which create an imbalance.

Each person should discuss his/her circumstances with their physician. Questions your physician may ask: How severe are your symptoms? What is your family history? What is your personal medical history? What are your goals? If you are feeling well and all parameters are good, consider why you want hormonal therapy? What is the end point of treatment? What are the alternatives and how effective are they compared to replacement therapy? To state that everyone going through menopause needs hormonal therapy would be premature. However, to mandate that no one could benefit from HRT would be short sighted.

*Cortisol: There are two major categories of stress hormones known as glucocorticoids (steroid stress hormone) and catecholamines. In humans, the two major stress hormones that represent each category are cortisol (glucocorticoid) and adrenaline (catecholamine). Both of these hormones play an important role in helping people respond appropriately to stressful situations such as injuries, illnesses and emotional situations. The hormone cortisol is often measured in individuals complaining of fatigue, weight loss or weight gain, or issues with blood sugar levels.

Cortisol is a hormone produced primarily by the adrenal glands. These glands sit on top of the kidneys or renal organs.

Cortisol, like the thyroid hormone, is also regulated by the pituitary gland in the brain.

A hormone called ACTH is released from the pituitary and interacts with the adrenal glands to regulate the production of cortisol. In acute stressful situations, these hormones support each other by preparing the body for potential action. In the initial phase of a stressful response, the levels of both chemicals increase. As a result, three reactions take place in the body:

1. Cells release glucose (sugar) from storage to be used for energy for the brain and muscles (including the heart);
2. A patient's heart rate and blood pressure increase to supply blood with nutrients to the important organs and structures such as the heart and muscles;
3. Blood is diverted away from intestines to supply other vital organs (after all digestion and absorption can utilize a fair amount of energy that would be better utilized elsewhere).

In the short term, this is a very helpful response system because it makes us more alert and prepared to respond. However, prolonged, untreated stress can have significant negative impact on our health and hormone levels. If cortisol levels remain elevated for an extended period of time, this can have adverse effects on the body, such as elevated blood sugar levels potentially increasing the risk of Type 2 diabetes, elevated blood pressure, weight gain, excess bruising, osteoporosis, and loss of short term memory. If your cortisol level is significantly elevated, your physician may evaluate you for Cushing's syndrome, a disease caused by the overproduction of cortisol in the body due to a tumor in the adrenal glands or malfunction of the brain's pituitary gland.

A deficiency of the cortisol hormone is equally as concerning to physicians. This condition is known as Addison's, a rare disease that occurs in one out of every 100,000 people. It occurs when the adrenal glands cannot produce sufficient cortisol. Cortisol helps to maintain blood pressure, regulate blood sugars and protein levels, regulate the immune system, as well as promote a sense of well-being and alertness. A lack of this hormone can cause problems with low blood sugar (hypoglycemia), low blood pressure, and inappropriate immune system response and fatigue.

It's important to remember that reviewing hormone evaluations, assessments and treatments are more about balance than absolute numbers. Pairing symptoms with laboratory test results along with lifestyle and other risk factors gives the wellness physician an opportunity to design the best treatment plan for each individual.

***

UPDATE

Kate's symptoms included poor sleep, weight gain, irritability and depression. She was self-medicating with food, coffee and soda to improve her moods and get an energy boost throughout the day. Considering Kate's long-standing history of poor diet, consumption of carbonated beverages and family history, a DEXA scan was ordered. It showed osteopenia (the beginning of loss of bone density). She also reported that her menstrual cycle was becoming irregular, even though the results of her annual visits to her gynecologist were normal.

Kate's age, coupled with her lifestyle and symptoms (insomnia, low libido, moodiness, menstrual irregularity and high stress) clearly called for a comprehensive hormone panel and a neurotransmitter evaluation. Her cortisol levels were measured at four points throughout the day. Her levels of testosterone, estrogen, progesterone and thyroid hormones were checked, along with the levels of neurotransmitters in her urine.

I suspected that Kate's lack of energy, moodiness and weight gain was also exacerbated by deficiencies of certain key nutrients. A comprehensive blood test that evaluated the body's nutrient deficiencies and needs was performed. Wellness medicine recognizes that replacing required nutrients is an integral part of putting the body back into balance and optimizing its function. However, overloading the body with nutrients it does not need may not be beneficial and even worse, may place an undue strain on the body, putting it even more out of balance. In my opinion, balance allows the restorative powers of the body to function, while imbalance promotes the disease process.

Kate's evaluation revealed that her thyroid registered a borderline normal value indicating it may not be functioning optimally. Her cortisol level was mildly elevated at all four test points. Stress and high cortisol levels can adversely affect the function of the thyroid. A high cortisol level can also cause an increase in blood sugar, and subsequently, insulin levels. This may increase the risk of Type 2 diabetes. High stress and high cortisol levels may have also contributed towards high blood pressure.

Kate's laboratory evaluation revealed an elevated fasting insulin level of 27, a slightly elevated HbA1c of 5.8 and fasting blood sugar level of 102. Given her family history and high blood pressure, a VAP study was performed. It revealed LDL level of 140 (high), HDL of 45 and triglyceride level of 180 (high). Her hs-CRP was 4 (slightly elevated). Kate's history combined with clinical test results indicated that she was at an increased risk for diabetes and atherosclerosis (formation of plaque in the arteries). Her screening EKG was normal so a baseline stress test was performed to look for signs of significant blockage in the arteries of the heart; this study was normal.

All of the test results indicated that Kate's stress levels and diet were adversely affecting her health.

Simple STEP 2
Choosing the Right Foods

With a medical assessment completed, it is time to start building a solid foundation for long-term health with disease-fighting foods and a nutritious diet. If you have elevated risk factors for heart disease, osteoporosis or even a hormonal imbalance, you can thank Mother Nature for providing the perfect balance of foods to help support your journey to wellness. Hippocrates is credited for saying, "Let food be your medicine, and medicine, your food." We should not take this phrase to mean that we should never use medications, but realize there is no drug or herb that replaces a solid nutritional and lifestyle foundation. Food is one of the most potent interventions – it can harm us or help us. Almost any medical intervention designed to lower the risk for developing chronic illnesses and accelerated aging can be enhanced with appropriate nutritional input.

Is incorporating a good nutritional base an all-or-nothing phenomenon? Do we go completely organic, or do we make gradual changes? If a person's diet consists of fast food, carbonated sodas and sugars, it may be best to take the time to become educated about the value of consuming more nutritious foods first, before insisting on purely organic choices. This is not to say that eating organic is not valuable. It simply means that everyone has his/her own individual path to optimal health and wellness.

Every time you visit the grocery store, your food choices give you an opportunity to greatly reduce your risks of developing cancers, such as breast, ovarian, uterine and prostate, as well as cardiovascular disease, stroke and diabetes. You have the opportunity to look younger, have healthier-looking skin, and reduce free radical damage that can accelerate the aging process. Once you truly understand the power and knowledge of healthy foods, you will never look at blueberries or broccoli the same way again.

Many of us have heard of the term antioxidant and know that foods high in antioxidants can help us stay healthy and may even help decrease risk of chronic diseases like heart disease, Type 2 diabetes and strokes. But what are antioxidants and how do we measure a food's antioxidant capacity? First, antioxidants are substances that reduce the damage caused by the waste products produced in the body during normal cellular function. Our cells carry out a series of reactions every day to keep our bodies fueled and running smoothly. During this process, unstable byproducts are created and must be neutralized and removed. If left unchecked or allowed to build up, these byproducts can cause significant damage to tissues and organs.

Antioxidants also play an important role in minimizing cellular damage. According to the USDA, the development of various chronic and degenerative diseases, along with neuronal degeneration diseases such as Alzheimer's and Parkinson's, and the aging process may be attributed to oxidative stress.

If antioxidants are so important, then how do we measure the antioxidant value of foods so we know we are on the right track? The "ORAC" (or Oxygen Radical Absorbance Capacity) database was developed by the USDA to measure the antioxidant ability of a particular food—that is, the food's ability to prevent free radicals, toxins, chemicals and pollutants from attacking healthy cells in the body. Foods with high ORAC values have a greater ability to slow the oxidative

processes and reduce free radical damage that can contribute to these age-related diseases and degeneration. Keep in mind this is one way to measure antioxidant value of foods. The antioxidant values of any given food can vary widely by region, harvesting process, and growing conditions.

The ORAC database places spices such as cinnamon, turmeric, basil and oregano at the top of the list. Unsweetened cocoa (used to make chocolate) ranked at the top of the list. Fruits such as apples, plums, blueberries and cranberries also ranked high. Of course no list would be complete without vegetables such as beets, broccoli, cauliflower, green peppers, carrots and tomatoes. (A complete listing of foods and their ranking is included in the appendix at the back of this book).

Specific compounds isolated from fruits and vegetables have been shown to have additional benefits. For example, berries contain a substance called anthocyanin. In several studies, anthocyanin extract has been shown to lower cholesterol naturally and may help lower risk of heart disease. Studies suggest that berries could potentially:

- Prevent the growth of cancer cells
- Reduce the risk of cardiovascular disease
- Improve eye function
- Limit oxidation damage to DNA
- Enhance glucose tolerance

Cranberries are known for preventing urinary tract infections because they block bacteria like E. coli from sticking to walls of the urethra and bladder. However, many people do not know that cranberries may also help fend off ulcers in a similar way. The berry concentrate prevents H. pylori bacteria from adhering to the stomach wall lining.

Black currants have been found to enhance the synthesis of nitric oxide that relaxes the aorta and other blood vessels, possibly supporting healthy blood pressure. These berries may also support the immune system's response to pathogens, potentially improving one's immunity to infections, and have been shown to stop the growth of many harmful bacteria.

The power of pomegranates is so strong that consumption actually begins the "death" of cancer cells in the prostate, colon, lung, breast and other cancers. Pomegranates may also help to reduce the inflammatory proteins and enzymes that damage cartilage in our joints. This may offer some protection to those prone to arthritic conditions. Research indicates that this fruit may also have a positive effect on cardiovascular health.

Greek yogurt is another great food to add to your breakfast menu because it contains lactobacilli, the healthy bacteria that may delay the onset of cancer (*Journal of the National Cancer Institute.* 1980 Feb; 64(2):263-5). Lactobacilli have also been found to have an inhibitory effect on human bladder cancer cells (*Journal of Urology.* 2002 Nov; 168(5):2236-9).

Another great food, especially for vegetarians, is tempeh. It is typically found in the refrigerated section of most grocery stores, alongside other vegetarian proteins. Tempeh is made from soybeans processed in a manner similar to cheese making. The soybeans are cracked and inoculated with a beneficial bacterium, then fermented and formed into flat blocks. Sometimes whole-grains like barley, brown rice or millet are added. Tempeh has a meaty texture and is often used as a meat substitute in cooking. It can be marinated or grilled and added to stews, soups and pasta sauces. It is high in protein (three ounces, or approximately one half cup, contains 16 grams of protein and no cholesterol), fiber and isoflavones. Isoflavones are phytoestrogens that have been shown to help reduce estrogen-induced cancers by blocking the body's natural estrogen (*Cancer Invest.* 2003; 21(5):744-57). Tempeh also has antioxidant properties and is potentially useful in lowering existing cholesterol levels. (Panum Institute in Copenhagen (*Am.J. Clin. Nutr.* 69, 1999, p. 419-25).

Tomatoes contain one of the world's most concentrated sources of lycopene. Studies show a strong association between the increased consumption of tomatoes and a lowered risk of certain cancers. Lycopene is best absorbed from tomatoes that are cooked, like tomato sauce. Enjoy them with a vegetable omelet for breakfast or add them to any salad or meal.

Ground flaxseeds should be a staple in any home. They are a source of lignans, which appears to prevent estrogen dominance in two ways. By attaching to excess estrogen receptor sites in the body, lignans make the receptor sites inaccessible to receive excess estrogen. Also, lignans may increase a protein called the sex binding hormone globulin (SBHG) that helps to remove excess sex hormones from circulation. Researchers at Duke University also found evidence to support the inhibition of prostate cancer by consuming flaxseeds. Some studies suggest that flaxseed may even support healthy cholesterol levels and reduce the risk of cardiovascular disease. As with anything else, moderation is key.

Adding garlic and onions to your diet may also reduce your risk of cancer. Garlic has been shown to inhibit the growth rate of breast and prostate cancer cells. Other vegetables packed with antioxidants are carrots, sweet potatoes and squash. A scientist at John Hopkins University is credited with discovering a compound abundant in broccoli sprouts called sulphurophane. This compound was shown to significantly reduce the risk of developing cancer, possibly by supporting the body's natural detoxification system and enhancing its ability to clear substances that can potentially cause DNA damage.

Foods That Support Muscle

Protein is the actual raw construction material for body cells – like bricks used for building. Body structures made from protein include skin, hair, nails, bones, connective tissue and muscle. Next to water, protein is the most abundant substance in your body, making up approximately 15-20 percent of your weight. Protein plays a role in the following functions:

- Building and repairing muscle tissue, organs, bones and connective tissue
- Enhancing moods through formation of neurotransmitters
- Helping to control appetite and cravings
- Potentially enhancing the immune system so we are better able to fight off infections
- Transporting oxygen throughout the bloodstream to organs and muscles.

Consuming sufficient amounts of protein at every meal is critical for the body to function optimally and may help weight loss and fitness efforts. If you eat protein at every meal, you feel fuller quicker. Protein is essential in building muscle. Muscle keeps your body burning fat more efficiently throughout the day. The more muscle you have, the more calories you burn at rest or when doing something passive, such as reading this book. When you exercise or lift weights, you break down muscle fibers, and protein helps repair and fortify muscles, and is required to build new muscle fibers.

How to Choose Healthy Protein

Protein comes from many food sources including beef, chicken and turkey, fish, and other seafood; as well as nuts and legumes including beans, lentils, peas, peanuts and soybeans (such as tempeh or tofu). You need to consume approximately ½ gram of protein for every pound of lean body weight on a daily basis. Keep in mind that this value is primarily for relatively sedentary individuals. For example, if you weigh 140 pounds, you would need 70 grams of protein per day. Examples of healthy protein choices include:

- 4 ounce chicken breast or salmon filet (28 grams protein)
- 1 cup cottage cheese (28 grams of protein)
- 1 egg with yolk (6 grams protein)
- 1 scoop whey protein (16-20 grams protein)
- 1 ounce almonds (6 grams protein)
- 1 tablespoon almond butter (4 grams protein)

A 4-ounce broiled porterhouse steak serves up 28 grams of protein, but also delivers 22 grams of fat, with nine grams of saturated fat. The same amount of salmon gives you 28 grams of protein and 9 grams of fat, with only 1.5 grams of saturated fat. A cup of cooked lentils has 18 grams of protein, but less than 1 gram of fat.

The best animal protein choices are fish and poultry. If you are partial to red meat, such as beef, pork, or lamb, stick with the leanest cuts, choose moderate sized portions, and consume only as an occasional part of your diet. Turkey is one of the leanest meat sources available and contains 1/3 of your daily requirement for niacin and vitamin B_6. Dark meat is a good source of iron and zinc. Avoid the self-basting turkeys because they have been injected with fat. Roast a turkey on Sunday, and you will have plenty of good-quality protein handy for a meal any day of the week.

Cutting down on saturated fat is easier to do when you eat tuna or salmon. You also benefit from a healthy dose of omega-3 fatty acids. These essential fatty acids have been shown to reduce inflammation throughout the entire body, and essential to relieving or combating depression.

Vegetable sources of protein, such as beans, nuts, and even whole grains, are excellent choices because they offer healthy fiber, vitamins and minerals. Nuts like almonds and cashews are a great source of healthy fat.

HEALTHY FATS AND DIGESTION: GOOD VS. BAD FATS

There are four major types of fats:

- Monounsaturated fats
- Polyunsaturated fats
- Saturated fats
- Trans fats

Monounsaturated fats and polyunsaturated fats are known as the "good fats" because they are good for your heart, cholesterol levels and overall health. Here are some examples to add to your diet, as indicated in Table 1.

Table 1: Good Fats

GOOD FATS	
Monounsaturated fat	**Polyunsaturated fat**
• Avocados • Nuts (almonds, peanuts, macadamia nuts, hazelnuts, pecans, cashews) • Olives • Peanut butter • Vegetable oils: canola, olive	• Cold-water, fatty fish: herring, mackerel, salmon, sardines, trout and tuna • Seeds: flax, pumpkin, sesame and sunflower • Soy products: soymilk, tempeh, tofu • Walnuts • Vegetable oils: corn, safflower and soybean

Saturated fats and all trans fats are labeled "bad fats" because they increase your risk of disease and elevate cholesterol levels. These fats tend to be solid at room temperature (think of butter or traditional stick margarine), while monounsaturated and polyunsaturated fats tend to be liquid (think of olive or corn oil).

Table 2: Bad Fats

BAD FATS	
Saturated fat	**Trans fat**
• Chicken with the skin • High-fat cuts of meat (beef, lamb, pork) • Lard • Palm and coconut oils • Whole-fat dairy products (butter, cheese, cream, milk, ice cream)	• Candy bars • Fried foods (French fries, fried chicken, chicken nuggets, breaded fish) • Commercially-baked pastries, cookies, doughnuts, muffins, cakes, pizza dough • Pre-packaged snack foods (crackers, microwave popcorn, chips) • Stick margarine • Vegetable shortening

General Guidelines for Choosing Healthy Fats

With so many different sources of dietary fat—some good and some bad—the choices can get confusing. The bottom line is simple:

Don't go no-fat– go good fat.

If you are concerned about your weight or heart health, rather than avoiding fat in your diet, try replacing saturated and trans fats with "good fats." This might mean replacing some of the meat you eat with beans and legumes, removing skin and fats from meats, or using olive oil rather than butter.

How much fat is too much?

Defining how much fat is too much in your diet depends on your lifestyle, your weight, your age, and most importantly your state of health. The USDA recommends that the average individual follow these guidelines:

- Keep total fat intake to 20-35 percent of total daily caloric intake.

- Limit saturated fats to less than 10 percent of your calories (200 calories for a 2,000 calorie diet).

- Limit trans fats to 1 percent of total daily calories consumed (2 grams per day for a 2,000 calorie diet).

How to Go from Bad to Good Fat

There are three simple things to remember about switching from bad to good fats.

- **Eliminate trans fats from your diet.** Check food labels for trans fats. Avoiding commercially processed or baked goods. Also limit your consumption of fast foods.
- **Limit your intake of saturated fats.** Cut back on red meat and full-fat dairy foods. Replace red meat with fish poultry, beans and nuts whenever possible, and switch from whole milk and other full-fat dairy foods to lower fat versions.
- **Eat omega-3 fats every day.** Good sources include fish, walnuts, ground flax seeds and flaxseed, canola or soybean oil.

Eliminating Trans Fats

A trans fat is a normal fat molecule that has been twisted and deformed during a process called *hydrogenation*. During this process, liquid vegetable oil is heated and combined with hydrogen gas. Partially hydrogenating vegetable oils makes them more stable and less likely to spoil– very good for food manufacturers but very bad for you. Remember: no amount of trans fats is healthy for the body and contribute to several major health problems – from heart disease to cancer.

Sources of Trans Fats

Many people think of margarine when they hear the word trans fats, and it's true that some margarine brands are loaded with them. However, the primary source of trans fats in the Western diet comes from consuming commercially prepared baked goods and snack foods. Baked goods, fried foods, solid fats semi-solid vegetable shortening and most stick margarines; boxed mixes (pancake, cake and chocolate drinks); snack foods like potato, corn, and tortilla chips, candy, and packaged or microwave popcorn are often loaded with trans fats.

Become A Trans Fat Detective

To ensure that you are buying the healthiest food possible, you need to become a detective when you shop. Manufacturers have become very smart "hiding" sugars and other additives and preservatives in seemingly "healthy" foods. Here are some tips to discover what's really inside your food.

- When shopping, read the labels and watch out for "partially hydrogenated oil" listed in the ingredients. Even if the food claims to be trans-fat free, this ingredient makes it suspect.
- With margarine, choose the soft-tub versions, and make sure

the product has zero grams of trans fat and contains no partially hydrogenated oils.

- When eating out, skip fried foods, biscuits, and other baked goods. Avoid these products unless you know that the restaurant has eliminated trans fat. Ask what type of oil your food will be cooked in.

- Avoid fast food. Most states have no labeling regulations for fast food, so they may contain hidden sources of trans fats.

Reducing Intake of Saturated Fats

When focusing on healthy fats, a good place to start is reducing your consumption of saturated fats. Saturated fats are mainly found in animal products such as red meat and whole milk dairy products. Poultry and fish also contain saturated fat, but in less amounts than red meat. Other sources of saturated fat include tropical vegetable oils, such as coconut oil and palm oil.

Simple Ways To Reduce Saturated Fat

- Eat less red meat (beef, pork, or lamb) and more fish and chicken.
- Remove the skin from chicken and trim as much fat off the meat as possible before cooking.
- Go for lean cuts of meat, and stick to white meat (which has less saturated fat).
- Avoid frying food and opt for baking, broiling, or grilling.
- Avoid breaded meats and vegetables and deep-fried foods.
- Choose almond or soymilk instead of whole milk.
- Use liquid vegetable oils such as olive or canola, instead of lard, shortening, or butter.
- Avoid cream and cheese sauces, or have them served on the side.

Here are some additional healthier options to reduce saturated fat in your diet, as illustrated in Table 3

Sources of Saturated Fats	Healthier Options
Butter	Olive oil
Cheese	Low-fat or reduced-fat cheese
Red meat	White meat chicken or turkey
Cream	Low-fat milk or fat-free creamer
Eggs	Egg whites, an egg substitute (e.g. Eggbeaters), or tofu
Ice cream	Frozen yogurt or reduced fat ice cream
Whole milk	Skim or 1% milk
Sour cream	Plain, non-fat yogurt

Consuming Healthy, Unsaturated Fats in Your Diet

Now that you know how to avoid saturated fat and trans fat, how do you add the healthy monounsaturated and polyunsaturated fats to your diet? The best sources are found in fish, nuts, seeds and vegetable oils, but you may also opt for these options:

- **Cook with olive oil**. Use olive oil rather than butter, stick margarine or lard. For baking, try canola or vegetable oil. Limit your use of refined oils and do not super heat any oils (avoid frying, for example) since they can produce damaging free radicals.
- **Eat more avocados.** Try them in sandwiches or salads or make homemade guacamole. Avocados are packed with

fats that are good for the heart and brain, and make a filling and satisfying meal. Approximately one-quarter of an avocado equals one serving size.

- **Reach for the nuts.** You can add nuts to vegetable dishes or use them instead of breadcrumbs on chicken or fish. To measure a serving size of nuts or seeds, they should cover no more than three outstretched fingers when spread flat across your hand.
- **Snack on olives.** Olives are high in healthy monounsaturated fats. Unlike most other high-fat foods, they make a great low-calorie snack. Try them plain or make a tapenade for dipping vegetables or whole-wheat crackers.
- **Dress your own salad**. Commercial salad dressings are often high in saturated fat or made with trans fat oils, as well as thickeners, salt, sugar, preservatives and other additives. Create your own healthy and tastier dressings with high-quality, cold-pressed olive oil, flaxseed oil or sesame oil.

Damaged Fat: When Good Fats Go Bad

A good fat can become bad if heat, light, or oxygen damages it. Polyunsaturated fats are the most fragile. Oils high in polyunsaturated fats (such as flaxseed oil) **must** be kept refrigerated in an opaque container. Cooking with these oils also damages the fats. Never use oils, seeds or nuts after they begin to smell or taste bitter. Heating oils to their smoking point makes them susceptible to damage.

Omega-3 Fatty Acids: Super Fats for The Brain and Heart

Omega-3 fatty acids are one type of polyunsaturated fat. While all types of monounsaturated and polyunsaturated fats are good for you, omega-3 fats are vital for normal metabolism. Your body cannot make them and must obtain them through food.

Omega-3s are essential for proper metabolism and retinal function, and have several other benefits, including:

- Prevent and reduce symptoms of depression
- Protect against memory loss and dementia
- Reduce the risk of heart disease, stroke, and cancer
- Ease arthritis, joint pain, and inflammatory skin conditions
- Support a healthy pregnancy
- Lower cholesterol and triglyceride levels
- Inhibit platelet clotting
- Reduce inflammatory and immune reactions

Omega-3 Fatty Acids and Mental Health

Omega-3 fatty acids are highly concentrated in the brain and play a vital role in cognitive function (memory, problem-solving abilities, etc.) as well as emotional health. Getting more omega-3 fatty acids in your diet can help you battle fatigue, sharpen your memory, and balance your mood. Studies have shown that omega-3s can be helpful in the treatment of depression, attention deficit/hyperactivity disorder (ADHD), and bipolar disorder.

There are three types of omega-3 fatty acids:

- **EPA and DHA** – Eicosapentaenoic acid (EPA) and docosahexaenoic acid (DHA) have the most research to back up their health benefits. Both are found in abundance in cold-water fatty fish, which obtain the fatty acids by consuming microalgae or plankton.
- **ALA** – Alpha-linolenic acid (ALA) comes from plants. Studies suggest that this omega-3 is a less potent form than EPA and DHA. The best sources come from flaxseed, walnuts, and canola oil.

Fish: The Best Food Source of Omega-3 Fatty Acids

The best sources of omega-3 fatty acids are cold-water, fatty fish such as salmon, herring, mackerel, anchovies, and sardines, or high-quality fish oil supplements. Canned albacore tuna and lake trout can also be good sources, depending on how the fish were raised and processed.

Some people avoid seafood because they worry about consuming mercury or other possible toxins in fish. However, most experts agree that the benefits of eating two servings a week of these cold-water fatty fish outweigh the risks. If you're a vegetarian or you don't like fish, you can still get your omega-3 fix by eating algae (which is high in DHA) or taking a fish oil or microalgae supplement.

Choosing the Best Omega-3

With so many omega-3 and fish oil supplements and fortified foods on the market, making the right choice can be tricky. These guidelines can help.

- **Avoid products that don't include the source of Omega-3s.** Does the package list the source of omega-3 fatty acids? If not, chances are it is ALA (sometimes from plain old canola or soybean oil), which most of us already get plenty of. ALA has not been shown to have the same cardiovascular benefits as long-chain essential fatty acids (DHA or EPA), and the body is ineffective at converting ALA to its more useful counterparts.
- **Don't fall for fortified foods.** Many fortified foods (such as margarine, eggs, and milk) claim to be high in omega-3 fatty acids, but the real amount of omega-3 is often miniscule.
- **Look for the total amount of EPA and DHA on the label.** The bottle may say 1,000 milligrams of fish oil, but it's the amount and types of omega-3 fatty acids that matter. Read the small print. It may show only 300 mg of EPA and DHA

(sometimes listed as "omega-3 fatty acids"), which means you need to take three capsules to get close to 1,000 milligrams of omega-3s.

- **Choose supplements that are mercury-free, pharmaceutical grade and molecularly distilled**. Make sure the supplement contains both DHA and EPA. Fish oil supplements can cause stomach upset and belching, especially when you first start taking them. To reduce these side effects, take the supplements with food. You may also want to start with a low dose and gradually increase it, or divide the dose among three meals.

How Much Omega-3 Do I Need?

The American Heart Association recommends consuming 1 to 3 grams per day of EPA and DHA (1 gram = 1,000 milligrams). For the treatment of mental health issues, including depression and ADHD, look for supplements that are high in EPA, which has been shown to elevate and stabilize mood. Aim for at least 1,000 milligrams of omega-3 fatty acids per day.

The Truth about Dietary Fat and Cholesterol

Cholesterol is a fatty, wax-like substance that your body needs to function properly. Cholesterol alone is not bad: however, when you consume too much, it can have a negative impact on your health.

Cholesterol comes from two sources: your body and food. Your body (specifically, the liver) produces some of the cholesterol you need naturally, but you also get cholesterol directly from any animal products you eat, such as eggs, meat and dairy. Together, these two sources contribute to your blood cholesterol level.

Good vs. Bad Cholesterol

Cholesterol is broken down into good and bad categories, depending upon the type of carrier molecule, or lipoprotein, transporting it through the bloodstream. Low-density lipoprotein is the bad type of cholesterol because it attaches to arterial walls, eventually building up and causing blockages. High-density lipoprotein (HDL) cholesterol is considered good because it binds with LDL and carries it to the liver to be removed from the body. The key to healthy cholesterol levels is to keep HDL high and LDL levels low.

Research shows that there is only a weak link between the amount of cholesterol you consume and actual blood cholesterol levels. The biggest influence on your total and LDL cholesterol is the *type* of fats you eat—not your dietary cholesterol. So instead of counting cholesterol, it's better to simply focus on replacing bad fats with good fats. Keep these tips in mind:

- Monounsaturated fats have been found to help lower total and bad (LDL) cholesterol levels, while increasing good cholesterol (HDL).
- Polyunsaturated fats lower triglycerides and fight inflammation.
- Saturated fats raise your LDL and total blood cholesterol levels.
- Trans fats are even worse than saturated fats, since they not only raise your bad LDL cholesterol, but also lower the good HDL cholesterol levels.

All cells, including those in the large intestine and your entire nervous system, require a constant influx of undamaged fatty acids and cholesterol to remain fully functional. If you don't ensure an adequate intake of healthy fats, your nervous system and the smooth muscles surrounding your digestive passageway that are responsible for creating peristaltic waves throughout your digestive tract may lose function.

Healthy fats are necessary for optimal absorption of fat-soluble vitamin A, which is critical to building and maintaining the mucosal lining of your colon.

Foods Rich in Healthy Fats Include:

- Avocados
- Coconut/coconut oil (although it is a saturated fat, if used in moderation, coconut appears not to adversely affect lipid levels and may promote reduction in abdominal obesity).
- Cold-water fish
- Extra-virgin olive oil
- Olives
- Organic eggs
- Raw nuts and seeds

Eat To Beat Depression

- Meat, fish, eggs, lentils and other sources of protein should be your culinary weapons of choice to beat the blues. Studies have shown that adding the amino acid tryptophan (one of the building blocks of protein) to the diets of people battling depression can improve moods.

- Eat more oily fish and nuts, too. The brain needs omega-3 fatty acids to perform properly. People who don't eat enough are more prone to depression.

- Whole grains—from oats to whole wheat bread—are great sources of complex carbohydrates that slowly release energy to prevent your blood sugar taking a nosedive, leaving you feeling downhearted.

- Fruits and vegetables are rich in zinc and folate, two nutrients that are important in helping to prevent depression.

- Cut out processed foods. People who eat fresh foods have much lower rates of depression.

Eat To Beat Brittle Bones

Diet remains important to bones in adulthood. One in two women and one in five men over the age of 50 will break a bone, mainly because of osteoporosis. Vitamin D_3 and calcium – dubbed "the sunshine vitamin" found in foods such as oily fish, milk and breakfast cereals – is essential in enabling your body to absorb calcium. You need 1,000 to 1,200 mg of calcium and 800 international units (IU) of vitamin D per day to decrease the risk of developing osteoporosis and Type 2 diabetes.

Good sources of calcium and Vitamin D come from a variety of foods including:
- Greek yogurt (low fat): one serving contains about 15 percent of one's daily requirement of calcium and 20 percent of the daily requirement of phosphorous, not to mention about 15 grams of protein. To make it even more nutritious, try adding fresh blueberries and a teaspoon of wheat germ (good source of B vitamins).
- Canned sardines with bones (one can provides about 35 percent of the daily calcium needed). Create a colorful, delicious meal by topping with chopped tomatoes and your favorite, low-fat salad dressing.
- Tofu: Add half-cup and stir fry with fresh vegetables.

- One cup cooked of bok choy provides about 74 mg of calcium. It is also a good source of a magnesium, phosphorous and potassium. You can also add to soups or grill this nutritious vegetable.

Vitamin K, found in foods such as broccoli, plays a role in moving the calcium from the arteries to the bones. Magnesium, found in chickpeas, nuts, lentils and potatoes, and lean sources of protein are also essential for building bone tissue.

Eat To Beat High Blood Pressure

Hypertension, or high blood pressure, is diagnosed when the systolic pressure (the top number) is 140 or above, and the diastolic pressure (the bottom number) is 90 or above. Lifestyle has a tremendous impact on high blood pressure—a healthy lifestyle can help you control your blood pressure and avoid, delay or reduce the need for medication.

According to a report published in 2011 by the Centers for Disease Control (CDC), most Americans consume too much salt and reducing our intake can help lower blood pressure. Federal guidelines announced in 2010 set the daily salt limit at 1,500 mg for African Americans, people ages 51 or older and people with high blood pressures, diabetes or chronic kidney disease; and at 2,300 mg for the rest of the U.S. population. The report also notes that about 75 percent of the salt in our diet comes from restaurant-prepared and commercial (packaged) foods. Consider cooking from scratch more frequently to reduce your sodium intake.

According to research by the Mayo Clinic, people who reduce their sodium consumption can lower blood pressure rates 2 to 8 mm Hg. Eating a diet rich in whole grains, fruits, vegetables and low-fat dairy products, as well as lower saturated fat and cholesterol, can also lower blood pressure up to 14 mm Hg. Fruits and vegetables with naturally occurring potassium can also support lower blood pressure.

The University of Maryland Medical Center cites the results of a clinical study of 8,500 women that found a higher intake of dietary magnesium may decrease the risk of high blood pressure. Foods rich in magnesium include whole grains (especially oatmeal), unsalted nuts, and green vegetables, especially green leafy varieties.

Eat To Beat Cancer

According to American Cancer Society's 2006 Guidelines on Nutrition and Physical Activity for Cancer Prevention, studies indicate that one third of cancer deaths in the U.S. are attributable to tobacco exposure and another third to diet and exercise habits. Maintaining a healthy weight tops the list of healthy lifestyle factors. Obesity is responsible for 14 percent of cancer deaths in men and 20 percent in women and continues to rise.

Most physicians agree that following a healthy, balanced diet, and eliminating tobacco and excessive alcohol consumption can prevent most cancers. Eating a healthy diet derived mostly from plant sources, including a variety of fruits, vegetables and whole grain products, provides nutrient extra protection with health-promoting nutrients and antioxidants. Some of the top foods include tomatoes, beans, onions and garlic, cruciferous vegetables (broccoli, cauliflower, cabbage, Brussels sprouts), dark leafy greens, berries, and whole grains.

Another recommendation is to limit alcohol consumption to less than one drink per day for women and two drinks per day for men. Just one drink a day increases the risk of certain cancers by 30 percent and has been linked to larynx, liver, pharynx, esophagus, mouth, colon, rectum and breast cancers.

Eat To Beat Low Energy

Nutrition experts agree that hydration has a large impact on our energy levels. People who ignore the thirst signal may experience nausea, loss of appetite, impaired physical performance and lower mental concentration. Long-term dehydration can lead to more serious complications. The Dietary Reference Intakes (DRI), **which offers nutrition** recommendations from the **Institute of Medicine** (IOM) of the U.S. **National Academy of Sciences**, suggests men should consume an average of 12 cups of fluid daily in order to stay well hydrated, while women should consume about nine cups per day. Even slight dehydration may leave you tired and lethargic so drinking water throughout the day is recommended.

Eating regular meals keeps blood sugar and energy levels steady. A breakfast that is high in fiber and protein will support mental concentration and satiety throughout the morning and help to control appetite. Smaller, lighter meals and snacks every three to four hours helps to prevent the dreaded afternoon energy slump. Two **to three servings of lean protein each day** prevents major fluctuations in blood glucose levels after eating high-carbohydrate foods, and may support a neurotransmitter balance that enhances alertness.

Go Nuts for Health

Eating nuts can help stabilize blood sugar levels and prevent health related complications. They are loaded with nutrients and support good health as long as they are eaten in moderation and unsalted. Eating two ounces of nuts daily in place of carbohydrates may be effective in controlling blood sugar and cholesterol levels in Type 2 diabetics. A variety of unsalted nuts, either raw or dry-roasted may be used as part of a strategy to improve diabetes without additional weight gain. The best choices include raw almonds, pistachios, walnuts, pecans, hazelnuts, peanuts, cashews, and macadamias.

Following these eating tips every day will leave you with a continuous supply of energy and mental clarity. You will notice the change immediately!

UPDATE:

It was clear that Kate's diet was a major contributor to her lack of energy and also played a role in her other symptoms. Kate needed to be educated and empowered about making better choices to improve her health and learn how to combat low energy levels, high blood pressure and brittle bones. One clear source of Kate's low energy came from not eating breakfast. The solution: she needed an easy and portable option. A balanced breakfast can be as easy as making a shake with protein powder, ground flaxseeds or oatmeal, blueberries (or any other berries), almonds, water or soymilk and a dash of cinnamon.

We embarked on a program to make Kate aware of the hidden ingredients, such as sodium and trans fats, in the fast foods she consumed on a regular basis. She was encouraged to eat fish high in omega-3 fatty acids, such as salmon, twice a week while incorporating other omega-rich foods such as walnuts, avocados and almonds in moderation. By focusing on adding foods such as kale and other green leafy vegetables, fresh fruits, low-glycemic grains and lean proteins to her diet, Kate was able to keep her energy levels high and lose weight.

Simple STEP 3
Why Healthy Digestion Is So Important

Healthy digestion is an important part of any anti-aging program. In the previous chapter, we talked about the amazing benefits that foods have on our health and well-being. However, in order to maximize these benefits, we have to be able to digest and absorb as many nutrients as possible from these foods. As we get older, our body's ability to produce the natural chemicals that aid digestion diminishes. This can contribute to compromised absorption, nutrient deficiencies and the potential worsening of conditions like anemia and chronic issues such as allergies and osteoporosis. Other factors that can interfere with proper digestion include certain medications, choosing foods that are low in natural enzymes, and experiencing extreme stress for a prolonged period.

To better understand how digestion influences our health, we must first get a better understanding of the normal digestive process. Digestion actually starts in the brain. Just the thought of food and the smell can stimulate the digestive process. The act of placing food in the mouth further stimulates digestive juices in the stomach and saliva production. Chewing provides the opportunity for food to combine with the saliva, which contains oral digestive enzymes. Saliva also contains a substance known as epidermal growth factor (EGF). This substance facilitates the healing of injured and inflamed intestinal tissue. Healthy tissue equals better absorption. While there is still some debate regarding how many times you should chew each bite, taking the time to chew foods properly may provide these benefits:

- Allows foods to be mixed with appropriate enzymes

to start digestive process.

- Prevents the fermentation of large chunks of food in the stomach, which can lead to symptom such as bloating, excess gas and reflux.
- Allows time for communication between the brain and the stomach and reducing chances of overeating.

Stomach

The next important step of the digestive process occurs when the food enters the stomach, stretches the stomach wall, and mixes with several substances that prepare the food for absorption. This secretion of gastrin causes the stomach cells to make hydrochloric acid, which activates the digestive enzyme called pepsin and changes the structure of proteins to allow pepsin to efficiently break them down into smaller molecules. If this process is compromised, then large protein molecules may enter into blood stream and create an abnormal immune response. Some physicians suggest that this is one of the underlying mechanisms contributing to conditions such as allergies and autoimmune dysfunctions. It is thought that hydrochloric acid may also have some other important functions including reducing bacterial overgrowth, helping with absorption of certain minerals, like calcium and zinc; and the extraction and absorption of iron from non-meat sources.

Why is hydrochloric acid important? One study found colonic bacteria (fecal bacteria) in the stomachs of up to 25 percent of people with low amounts of stomach acid. Talk about bad breath! Now imagine if the bacteria that were allowed to grow out of control. It could lead to infections. It could also lead to a decrease in the absorption of important nutrients like vitamin K, folic acid and magnesium. We know that vitamin K helps blood to clot properly. Recent studies suggest that vitamin K may also help to prevent fractures and may be important in combating vascular disease. Folic acid is important for healthy red blood cells, prevents neural defects in the fetus, and plays a pivotal role in supporting better moods.

As we get older, our production of hydrochloric acid may decrease and cause digestion problems. Other things that can affect the production of this important acid are conditions such as atrophic gastritis, the inappropriate or excessive use of antacids, and taking certain medications. Symptoms like bloating, indigestion, excess gas and even reflux can be caused by compromised hydrochloric acid production. If you are experiencing these symptoms consistently, your Wellness Physician may use additional diagnostic tools, such as Heidelberg pH testing to examine the stomach's pH before and during the digestive process. A lactulose hydrogen breath test may also be performed to determine if there is an overgrowth of bacteria in the upper intestinal tract. If your symptoms or history are suspicious, then your physician may refer you for an upper endoscopy to look for ulcers or significantly inflamed stomach or esophagus.

Another important function of a healthy stomach is the preparation of vitamin B12 for absorption into the small intestine. Vitamin B12 helps with the formation of healthy red blood cells and can support improved energy levels, focus and moods.

As food exits the stomach, it enters the small intestine where it combines with bile from the liver and gallbladder, plus digestive enzymes from the pancreas. Bile salts help with the absorption of fats and fat-soluble vitamins. Digestive enzymes break down proteins, fats and carbohydrates. During this process, foods are further prepared for optimal absorption. If digestive enzymes or bile is insufficient, then nutrients may not be absorbed properly and can contribute to deficiencies or disorders of the immune system. For example, bile helps with the preparation of fats for absorption in the intestine. If bile salts are not able to do their assigned jobs, this can lead to deficiencies or insufficient levels of essential fatty acids, such as omega-3 and fat-soluble vitamins, like vitamin A and E.

Small Intestine

The health of the wall of the small intestine plays a key role in digestion. Small finger-like projections along the wall increase the surface area available for nutrient absorption. The cells that comprise the wall are densely packed and have several mechanisms to ensure that only small nutrients can enter the blood stream. If larger sized nutrients pass through, the body may treat them as a foreign substance, activating the immune system. If this happens repeatedly, evidence shows that it may lead to a condition of the intestinal lining referred to as "leaky gut syndrome." This can lead to an over active immune system, intensifying allergies, exacerbating autoimmune responses and contributing to ongoing problems with abdominal bloating, excessive gas and cramps, fatigue, food sensitivities, joint pain, skin rashes, and autoimmunity. Integrative physician Dr. Andrew Weil notes that the causes of this syndrome may due to chronic inflammation, food sensitivity, damage from taking large amounts of non-steroidal anti-inflammatory drugs (NSAIDS), cytotoxic drugs, radiation or certain antibiotics; excessive alcohol consumption or compromised immunity.

Along the border of these intestinal villi are hydrolase enzymes that handle the final break down of polysaccharide sugars such as sucrose (table sugar) into the simple sugars glucose and fructose, known collectively as monosaccharides. Simple sugars are transported into the intestinal cells for absorption into the blood stream via capillaries. Transport of glucose into the cells is dependent on the sodium-potassium pump. Sodium binds and changes the pump in order to carry glucose. The pump then carries both sodium and glucose into the cells, which then adds sodium into the space between the cells. As the sodium level between the cells increases, water osmotically moves from the intestinal cavity, or lumen, back into blood vessels for recirculation. This decreases the amount of water lost by the body. Another transporter pumps glucose and other simple sugars into the space between cells, where they also enter into circulation for the body to convert to energy. Keep in mind that sodium (salt) helps sugar (glucose) to be absorbed more efficiently by the body. While the body does need glucose for energy, excess sugars are converted and stored as fats, and cause a host of other problems, as discussed earlier.

The digestion of protein also continues in the small intestine. For protein to be absorbed, it must be converted to very small molecules, such as amino acids (building blocks of protein) or dipeptides (precursors to amino acids). Just as there are enzymes on the wall of the small intestine for sugars, enzymes also exist for proteins. These enzymes, called proteases, include peptidases and proteinases. Sodium-dependent transporters pump the amino acids into the spaces between cells where they diffuse into blood vessels and move into circulation, a process similar to glucose processing.

Fats in diet need to be emulsified by bile that enters the small intestine from the gall bladder. During this process, the pancreatic enzyme lipase acts on the fats during the digestion process. If this emulsification process is diminished, a person can develop issues with digesting and absorbing fats appropriately. They may encounter an increase in bowel gas, abdominal bloating and even diarrhea. Also, remember that certain vitamins are fat soluble, so poor digestion or absorption of fats may cause deficiencies in fat-soluble vitamins. Individuals who have had their gall bladders removed may experience some of these symptoms. Medications, such as

Orlistat, used to treat obesity, decrease the effectiveness of the enzyme lipase and prevent the digestion and absorption of fats. This could result in deficiencies of essential vitamins A, D, E and K.

The digestion and absorption process is a well-coordinated symphony that depends on all systems functioning in a state of optimal health. Things that damage the intestinal surface and environment, such as excessive alcohol intake, imbalanced bacterial flora, medications such as steroids, and stress can manifest as abdominal problems and nutritional deficiencies. A study published in *The American Journal of Gastroenterology* found that stress exacerbated symptoms of inflammatory bowel diseases, such as ulcerative colitis, were higher than physical factors, such as anti-inflammatory medications or even infections.

Celiac and Crohn's diseases can also affect health of the small intestine. People with celiac disease are unable to process a gluten protein that naturally occurs in wheat, rye and barley, and found in consumer products like vitamins, medicines and cosmetics like lip balm. Celiac disease exposes the intestinal walls to gluten and triggers an immune response that destroys the villi of the intestinal wall. Since these villi play such an important role in the digestion and absorption processes, nutrient deficiencies often develop in untreated sufferers. Symptoms of celiac disease may include abdominal bloating, constipation, foul smelling stools, diarrhea and weight loss. Even conditions such as unexplained iron-deficient anemia, osteoporosis, joint pain, fatigue, depression, anxiety, rash and canker sores can be symptoms of this disease. Diagnosis is made through laboratory testing and/or biopsy of the small intestinal wall.

Large Intestine

After passing through the small intestine, food enters the large intestine where more water and electrolytes, such as sodium, are removed from the food. In the colon, bacteria help with the production of certain vitamins, such as K, B1 (thiamine) and B2 (riboflavin). Colonic bacteria also act on the non-digestible particles to create many substances, including short-chain fatty acids (SCFA), the primary source of food for the cells along the colon wall. One of these in particular, butyrate, has been shown to decrease the risk of colon cancer.

A study published in the journal *Intestinal Microbiology 2000* 1(2): 51-58, suggests that the metabolites (broken-down elements) of carbohydrates, such as SCFA, may be more beneficial than protein metabolites, such as ammonia and N-nitrosocompounds (NOC). In fact, metabolites of proteins may be toxic, and create carcinogenic effects on the colon. Non-digestible carbohydrates (fiber) decrease the production of some of these toxic substances. If you need another reason to increase your dietary fiber intake, a study published in *Carcinogenesis* found that diets high in meats and fats and low in fiber are associated with increased risk of colorectal cancer.

To optimize digestion and keep your stomach and bowel movements functioning and regular, here are 11 things you can do right now:

1. **Encourage friendly bacteria in the digestive tract.**
   Maintaining a healthy population of friendly bacteria in your digestive tract promotes optimal digestion and prevents harmful organisms (like bacteria, yeast, parasites and fungi) from multiplying and taking over. Healthy bacteria, also known as probiotics, can be found in fermented foods like yogurt, sauerkraut and kefir.

2. **Eat four to five small meals per day.**
   The American Gastroenterology Association recommends eating four to five smaller meals per day without increasing overall caloric intake. Eating a whole meal, rather than grazing, ensures that the stretch receptors in the stomach are stimulated, triggering normal and mass peristaltic (contractile) waves throughout your small and large intestines, thereby moving waste material through your colon and rectum. The wastes come together to form roundish masses called boluses. With proper meals the boluses become well-formed stools that are easily and comfortably eliminated from your body.

3. **Eat a diet rich in raw fruits, vegetables and fiber daily.**
   Fiber nourishes colonocytes, the cells of the colon, and may help prevent colorectal cancers. It also adds bulk to the boluses of waste material in the large intestine, enabling the colon to turn the waste materials into well-formed stools. Adequate fiber intake is easily maintained when one eats a diet rich in vegetables, fruits, legumes and whole grains.

   It is helpful to increase intake of raw fruits and vegetables because they are rich in nutrients, water and natural digestive enzymes. Good choices include apples, avocadoes, blueberries, blackberries, grapes, lemons, pears, pineapples, strawberries, and all vegetables. Spend some time in the produce section and make them a part of every meal.

4. **Do not overcook vegetables**. This destroys many of the nutrients and makes them lose their flavor. You may be surprised by the delicious flavors of properly cooked vegetables.

5. **Limit red meats, especially those cooked on an open flame**. Grilling meats has been linked with higher nitrate levels in the colon, which has been associated to an increased risk of colorectal cancer and diabetes.

6. **Avoid refined carbohydrates,** such as white flour products (certain cereals, crackers, breads and pastas) and refined sugar. These foods are low in fiber and can increase blood sugar and insulin levels too quickly.

7. **Take time to chew foods well.** This simple practice has several benefits. First, you are savoring and relishing every delicious morsel. Second, you are giving the gut and the brain time to communicate to avoid overeating. Even more importantly, this simple act leads to the release of a substance that helps with healing and repair of the digestive lining. Remember that digestion starts in the mouth.

8. **Ensure adequate intake of water and water-rich foods.** Water is absorbed throughout the entire length of the colon and helps move waste materials along their journey. Insufficient water intake can cause stools to form before waste materials reach the rectal pouch, which can cause constipation. If you consume adequate servings of water-rich plant foods, like lettuces and juicy fruits, your water requirements may be decreased. Otherwise, pay attention to your body's thirst signal and drink several glasses of water daily. However, do not drink too much liquid just before eating. Drinking liquids with your meals dilutes stomach acid making it difficult for your stomach to do its job – digest your food. One glass of water should suffice.

9. **Consider supplementing with digestive enzymes** that contain hydrochloric acid, which helps break down food. Again check with your doctor to be sure that your

symptoms do not represent ulcers of stomach or duodenum, which can be life threatening.

10. Exercise and manage stress.

The results of several studies support the notion that exercise helps reduce or eliminate gastrointestinal problems such as stomach pain, diarrhea and irritable bowel syndrome. The lack of exercise is one of the causes of constipation.

Yoga combines stress reduction and exercise, an effective combination for decreasing symptoms of irritable bowel syndrome and alleviating constipation. Yoga is also recommended by the National Heartburn Alliance as a low-impact exercise (along with bicycle riding and Pilates) that can reduce heartburn symptoms if done at least two hours after eating.

Stress has a negative impact on the nervous system and can interfere with digestion. In addition to practicing yoga regularly, a few deep-breathing exercises before meals can be a fantastic stress management tool. Try this simple breathing exercise: Close your eyes and inhale through the nose – hold it for a count of four, then exhale through the mouth for a count of four.

11. Eliminate when the urge comes.

When the urge to have a bowel movement is suppressed, waste materials spend more time than necessary in the colon, causing them to become dehydrated and turn into hard stools.

Quick Home Remedy for Indigestion
To resolve heartburn and indigestion, stir one teaspoon of apple cider vinegar in a glass of water and drink. It may burn going down initially, but you should feel relief within 20 minutes. If symptoms persist or worsen, you need to consult your doctor or gastroenterologist for further evaluation. Persistent inflammation of the esophagus may lead to an increase risk of esophageal cancer.

UPDATE:

One of Kate's persistent conditions was acid reflux. Her patterns of eating late and on the run were contributing factors to the issue. Also, it is widely accepted that many foods such as coffee, sodas and fried foods can exacerbate symptoms of reflux. Kate's gastroenterologist had performed an endoscopy before our visit, and the results showed no evidence of inflammation or ulceration in the stomach. A Heidelberg pH capsule test confirmed that Kate had insufficient acid in the stomach, possibly compromising her body's ability to digest and absorb proteins and other nutrients. This may have also contributed to Kate's low energy levels and made it challenging to build muscle mass. She was prescribed small doses of replacement betaine hydrochloric acid (stomach acid) to take with her meals to aid in the digestive process. With her change in diet and the addition of this supplement, her digestive symptoms were significantly reduced.

Simple STEP 4
Exercise – The BEST Anti-Aging Tool

If we could put all of the benefits of exercise into one pill, it would probably be the most effective anti-aging health remedy available. Imagine taking a pill that could improve your mood and libido, relieve stress, increase your energy levels, decrease your risk of diabetes and heart disease, help maintain a healthy weight, counteract the loss of muscle tone, improve balance and coordination, and enhance your ability to learn. Who wouldn't be first in line to get this pill? Well, line up, because even though it is not in a pill form, this miracle intervention is readily available.

Admittedly, it can be a challenge to incorporate exercise in our overly scheduled, hectic lives. The obstacles seem to be endless: "I don't have enough time." "I am too tired." "I hate the gym." "I am too overweight." "I'm too old." "I am too uncoordinated." "I have children." "I don't need to lose weight." "It's boring." The excuses go on and on...

The best way to overcome these challenges is to look at exercise in a different light and reframe it within the context of your life. Sometimes the goal of losing weight is simply not enough motivation to get moving. We may need to shift our focus; instead of viewing exercise as simply a weight loss tool, consider it as one of the best anti-aging and health tools at our disposal. Many people feel that if they cannot commit to at least one hour per day then they should not bother to do anything at all.

Yet, according to the American College of Sports Medicine, studies show that exercising for as little as ten minutes several times a day has cumulative benefits. If your goal is to improve where you are right now, then whatever activity you choose to do is taking the first steps to a healthier you!

So how do you start? First, find a way to incorporate exercise into your daily routine by finding an activity you enjoy doing. Keep in mind: this is not an "all or nothing" strategy. You can start by taking simple steps: take the stairs instead of the elevator; park at the far end of the parking lot so you are forced to walk a little farther each day; or get up from your desk several times a day to stretch or take a brief walk. The more you do, the better you feel; the better you feel, the more you do. Now, that is a nice cycle to start.

Exercise, Insulin and Leptin

For years, research has demonstrated that the benefits of exercise far exceed a simple equation of calories burned during activity. Exercise and movement, along with a healthy diet, has a direct effect on the endocrine system's ability to regulate hormones. Specifically, exercise has been shown to increase sensitivity to both leptin and insulin, two powerful hormones that influence how energy is metabolized throughout the body. Insulin transports glucose from the foods you eat into your cells, and regulates blood sugar. Leptin appears to regulate the body's energy usage through metabolism and appetite. Proper leptin levels give us the feeling of satiety (telling us when to stop eating) and signals the body to burn calories, rather than store them as fat.

Insulin and Leptin Resistance

Through complex reactions to many factors—including high fat, low-nutrient diets, stress, and a lack of exercise—the body can become resistant to these hormones. This means that the body needs higher and higher levels of leptin and insulin to respond to their signals, often leading to a distorted appetite, poor energy levels, and unwanted weight gain.

While the exact relationship between leptin and insulin is still being studied, leptin appears to play a role in modulating the pancreatic cells that release insulin, according to animal studies done at Harvard University's Joslin Diabetes Center. Insulin resistance means that the cells do not respond well to insulin, so insulin levels become higher and eventually blood sugar goes up as well. You can see why insulin resistance can lead to pre-diabetes and Type 2 diabetes. High insulin levels have also been linked to inflammation and increased risks for developing chronic diseases, such as heart disease, arthritis and osteoporosis.

Exercise Improves Leptin and Insulin Sensitivity

The first line treatment for insulin resistance is exercise and weight loss, often paired with a diet that maintains a low-glycemic index. Results from the Diabetes Prevention Program presented in the *New England Journal of Medicine* in 2002 showed that exercise and diet were nearly twice as cost effective as the anti-diabetic drug Metformin in reducing the risk of progressing from insulin resistance to Type 2 diabetes.

While research has shown that leptin-resistant obese animals and humans do not benefit from the administration of supplemental leptin alone, exercise may help to reverse leptin resistance, according to a University of Florida study. By studying both obese and normal weight lab rats that consumed a high-fat diet, researchers found combining modest exercise with leptin hormone therapy seemed to renew the hormone's ability to function properly. The combination worked to prevent weight gain, even though neither worked alone among the control rat groups. In addition, the amount of weight the animals kept off was proportional to how much they ran on a treadmill. Simply put, modest exercise may help leptin to work properly, resulting in reduced weight gain.

Interval training appears to have a particularly strong impact on the regulation of leptin and insulin. Short bursts of vigorous exercise interspersed throughout a moderate-level workout appear to have long-term positive effects on how these two key metabolic hormones are used in the body. Even though studies suggest that exercising 30 minutes five times a week is required to maximize the effect on improving insulin resistance, I am sure that most experts would agree any movement is better than no movement. A simple walking program with intervals of jogging can help start the shift of the body's leptin and insulin into their proper mode. With these hormones operating more efficiently, energy and appetite become well regulated.

The benefits of exercise are physical, mental and psychological. They include:

1. **Lowered blood sugar**. Studies show that exercise improves HbA1c (marker for diabetes control) and improves the body's response to insulin.

2. **Building muscle mass**. Muscle burns more energy faster than any other tissue. As you build muscle, you

can become a fat-burning–rather than fat-storing–machine.

3. **Lowers Cholesterol**. Studies show that exercise can reduce LDL (bad cholesterol) and it can boost the levels of HDL (good) cholesterol.

4. **Protects the Heart**. Exercise reduces the risk of stroke, heart attack or other cardiovascular problems including diabetes and lowers blood pressure.

5. **Produces "feel-good" chemicals in the brain**. Exercise releases endorphins, the brain chemicals that boost your mood and make you feel happy, as well as relieve stress, and enhance your self-esteem and self-confidence. Exercise has also been shown to increase neurotransmitters, such as serotonin and dopamine that help us feel and sleep better. Some studies suggest that exercise is as effective as prescription medicine when treating some forms of depression.

6. **Helps you look and feel better**. Gaining muscle and reducing body fat, as well as increased strength and energy, will make you noticeably look and feel better.

7. **Prevents constipation**. Exercise increases the contractions of the wall of the intestine, helping to move the stool through the intestinal tract easier, and decreasing the time it takes to pass through the large intestine. However, exercising too soon after eating can divert blood flow away from the gut and toward the muscles, weakening peristaltic contractions and slowing the movement of the stool. Bloating and increased flatulence can result. It is recommended to wait at least an hour or two after eating, before doing any vigorous

activity so that the intestinal walls have adequate blood flow for proper peristalsis. Drinking plenty of water is necessary to prevent dehydration since water and electrolytes are lost through sweating.

8. **Prevents brittle bones**. According to the National Osteoporosis Foundation, the best types of exercise to maintain bone strength are weight bearing—that is, any activity you do while on your feet and legs that works your muscles and bones against gravity. Examples include walking, jogging, dancing and yoga. Swimming and bicycling are considering non-weight bearing. During weight-bearing exercises, the bones adapt to the impact of the weight and the pull of muscles by building more bone cells, increasing strength and density and decreasing the risks of fractures, osteopenia and osteoporosis. Muscle strengthening exercises, such as weight-resistance training, also increases bone density and can help reduce the symptoms of numerous diseases and chronic conditions including arthritis.

9. **Regular, moderate exercise has also been shown to enhance immunity, while both sedentary behavior and overtraining lead to suppressed immunity.** Some proposed theories on how this occurs:

    a. Moderate exercise increases the rate at which antibodies flow through blood stream.
    b. The increased temperature generated during moderate exercise makes it difficult for certain infectious organisms to survive.
    c. Moderate exercise can decrease levels of stress hormones, while excessive exercise can decrease immunity and increase stress hormones, negatively affecting immunity.

There are many different types of exercise, each offering their own unique benefits. Aerobic exercise has been associated with improving cardiovascular health, improving immunity, improving blood pressure, improving endurance, increasing good cholesterol levels and reducing bad cholesterols, and may actually even help us live longer. In order to reap all of the benefits of aerobic exercise, it is recommended to do 150 minutes of moderate aerobic activity weekly (five sessions per week of 30 minutes each) or 75 minutes of vigorous activity per week (four sessions of 20 minutes each). Moderate activity includes brisk walking, mowing the lawn, swimming or riding a bike. Running and intense dancing would constitute vigorous activity.

Resistance training is now strongly recommended by the American Heart Association and the American College of Sports Medicine to improve health and fitness. Resistance training combined with aerobic exercise may enhance the benefits of a workout, such as improving insulin resistance and cardiac functions as well as modifying the level and ratio of cholesterol and other cardiovascular risk factors.

In addition, resistance training also offers some unique benefits such as helping to maintain bone strength, improving basal metabolic rate that regulates weight management, and improving muscle tone and function to preserve balance and function, especially as we get older. Incorporating resistance training two to three times per week for three to six months can increase muscle strength from 25 to 100 percent in individuals.

The recommended frequency of weight-resistance training is a minimum of twice per week by performing one set of eight to 10 repetitions in eight to 10 different muscle groups. Body resistance, bands, free weights such as wrist weights or barbells and machines can all be utilized in resistance training.

Beginners and individuals who have not worked out in a while should consider starting with resistance machines and using a trainer to minimize chance of injury. Older individuals prone to balance and equilibrium issues as well as joint and range of motion issues may also benefit by using resistance machines.

Stretching and flexibility training are also an important part of maintaining physical fitness and function. While stretching does not improve muscle strength or endurance, it plays an important role in preventing injuries, promoting relaxation and increasing range of motion of the joints.

With any exercise program, it is important to check with your physician to ensure that you are physically able to participate and choose the right intensity level. If you have issues with your joints or have had a joint replacement, for example, you may have range of motion limitations. Remember, the goal is to feel better, not to create an injury. Working initially with a certified physical trainer will help you safely and effectively perform each exercise and teach you how to modify each activity for your particular needs.

Yoga Anyone?

Yoga, a mind-body practice with origins in ancient Indian spiritual philosophy, combines exercises that utilize strength, flexibility and breathing. The various styles of yoga that people use for health purposes typically combine physical postures (asanas), breathing techniques (pranayama), and meditation or relaxation. There are many styles of yoga: hatha is the one most commonly practiced in the United States and emphasizes asanas and pranayama. Most yoga practitioners use yoga to achieve fitness, relaxation and mental clarity. Studies suggest that yoga may be helpful to improve strength and flexibility, manage stress, lower heart rate and blood pressure, and help manage depression, anxiety and insomnia.

Pilates Perfection

Pilates is a form of exercise that focuses attention on the core (abdominal) muscles. The practice trains the mind to build symmetry and coordination in the body, and all fitness levels can participate. Those who are consistent with Pilates notice improvements in their flexibility, circulation, range of motion, posture and abdominal strength, and lowered levels of back, neck and joint pain.

One of the key benefits of Pilates is stronger and flatter abdominal muscles, which builds a foundation for total body strength and balance. By creating a stronger, healthier back and body awareness, practitioners stand straighter, taller and gain greater flexibility. Pilates aims to change the body's shape, including a flatter midsection that maintains flexibility in the abdominal muscles so that the entire body feels balanced.

As you can see, the choices of exercise are as varied as the individual. So excuses are gone!

UPDATE:

Kate's life was relatively sedentary, and it was clear that instituting some form of exercise routine would provide health benefits and support her dietary changes. Starting with a routine of walking while carrying a light set of weights, Kate slowly noticed that she was losing weight and her energy levels improved. She also realized that she was feeling less tense and anxious. After initially working with a trainer, she discovered that cross training (combining aerobics with light weights) allowed her to consistently fit a good workout into her busy schedule. She found that this form of exercise allowed her to keep the length of her workouts to 20 to 30 minutes on the days when she had limited time.

With her improved energy levels, Kate explored Pilates, yoga, Zumba and even kickboxing as part of her exercise routine. She discovered that Pilates made her more conscious of her posture and incorporated flexibility and resistance training at the same time. She discovered that a variety of exercises helped her stay focused and avoid burnout. Kate was walking taller and enjoying her new strength, energy and figure. She even dusted off her roller blades.

Simple STEP 5
Stress Management

According to Harvard University researchers, stress accounts for 60 to 90 percent of visits to the doctors each year. Stress is linked to heart disease, depression, hypertension, diabetes, asthma, chronic pain, headaches and insomnia. However, if you asked many of these patients if they believe that stress contributed to their illness, many may respond with a resounding "NO!" But, if you asked questions such as: "How often do you feel anxious for no reason?" "Do you dread opening your eyes to start the day?" "Do you crave salty or sweet foods?" "Do you feel tired all the time, but have received a clean bill of health by your physician?" All these may be signs that your body cannot keep up with the demands placed on it.

What is stress? Is there "good" and "bad" stress? If there is good and bad stress, then how do we differentiate between them? Is every response to stress always bad? Most importantly, is there anything that can be done to limit the negative effects of prolonged stress?

First, let's attempt to define stress in simple terms. Stress is a series of reactions produced in the body by a physical, emotional or environmental trigger. These reactions are designed to create a split-second decision process called "fight or flight." For example, if it is an infection, the response is designed to fight the infection. If it is rabid dog, then hopefully the response is to run away like an Olympic sprinter. If a pending deadline is looming, many of us depend on the stress response to energize and motivate us to complete the project. Many times stress produces a beneficial response that is referred to as eustress (good stress). However, when the signal or trigger is prolonged, our bodies become stuck in overdrive, using up all of our resources and making our body and mind feel tired and weak. This response (often referred to as dis-stress) can increase our risk of chronic health issues.

Short-term vs. Chronic Stress
Believe it or not, short-term stress *helps* our bodies, prompting a fight-or-flight response from the nervous system that revs up our heart rate, blood pressure, breathing and even our sweat glands. It's what puts the "go" in our get-up-and-go, allowing us to accomplish tasks and get out of the way if something is threatening our safety.

Chronic stress is a different story. It puts the body's motor in constant overdrive, raising your risk for heart disease, diabetes, autoimmune disorders and even obesity. A study published in the journal *Homeostasis* showed that stress has a greater effect on cholesterol than diet alone. If we consider that our stress hormones are derived from cholesterol molecules, then you can see how an increased demand for stress hormones could correlate with greater cholesterol production by the body. Remember, a large percentage of cholesterol in the body is manufactured naturally in the body, and not solely obtained through food.

Mechanics of the Stress Response: The Brain's Response
Stress events are first registered by the brain, which asks, "Is this a threat?" "If this is a threat, then do I set off the alarm, and if so, how loud should it be?" Interpretation is based on many factors including previous experiences and emotional state of mind. Through a series of intricate neurochemical

reactions the brain communicates with the adrenal gland and the body to generate a series of responses designed to prepare the body for action.

The Role of Adrenal Glands

Many of us are aware that the adrenal glands play a major role in our stress response. The adrenal glands are two triangular shaped organs that sit on top of the kidneys or renal glands (the term adrenal meaning on top of renal). Commonly referred to as the "fight-or-flight" response system, the adrenal glands carry out the events designed to prepare the body to respond to the situation. This is done through two major stress chemical messengers: cortisol and adrenaline (hence the term "adrenaline rush"). The body responds in a series of steps in a matter of seconds: the adrenals increase blood sugar levels (to provide energy); the heart rate and blood pressure increase (to ensure blood flows to the vital organs like the brain, heart, muscles, etc.); blood flow to the gut decreases and is diverted to other areas where it is needed, such as the heart, lung and the muscles; and the pupils dilate to ensure maximum light input. All of these steps are necessary to prepare the body to fight or flee in an emergency.

However, an excessive activation of this system can have a negative impact on our health and well-being. If the stress system remains activated too long, it can lead to a chronic elevation of blood sugar and insulin levels, thereby increasing the risk of diabetes. Because cortisol helps to break down muscles to use for energy, prolonged exposure to cortisol can lead to the excessive break down of muscles in the extremities. Excess cortisol can also contribute to fat formation in the face and mid-section. We know now that truncal (abdominal) obesity contributes to increased inflammation and risk of heart disease, strokes and diabetes. Excess cortisol can also lead to increased production of stomach acid, which can lead to the formation of ulcers in the stomach, and decreased immunity allowing more frequent infections.

Cortisol and sex hormones share a common origin, so prolonged stress can affect sex hormones levels. Decreased production of hormones such as estrogen and testosterone can lead to symptoms of hormonal imbalance such as irregular periods, decreased libido and possible early menopause. Elevated cortisol and adrenaline levels can affect sleep patterns and cause insomnia. Several studies show that insomnia is an additional risk factor for obesity and the development of Type 2 diabetes. Stress can affect memory and destroy brain cells. As if that were not enough, excess cortisol can increase the rate serotonin (the neurotransmitter that helps you to feel good) is removed from the brain while decreasing the rate the neurotransmitter is formed. This can lead to increased feelings of depression and anxiety. Since serotonin also plays a role in controlling appetite, it is common for people to experience excessive cravings when they are stressed.

The excess cortisol generated by prolonged stress can also contribute to osteoporosis. First, excess cortisol inhibits the rate calcium is absorbed from the gut and decrease the activity of cells that help to form bone tissue (osteoblasts). The result is an increased risk of fractures.

Stress can also affect the function of the thyroid leading to weight gain, high cholesterol and decreased energy. Excess cortisol can prevent the proper release of the hormone from the brain (TSH) that stimulates the thyroid to make hormones and function normally.

Stress can also have a devastating effect on our ability to survive adversity such as a traumatic injury or severe illness.

The *Journal of the American Medical Association* published a study in 1992 that looked at the survival rate of people diagnosed with coronary artery disease, a condition that causes heart attacks. To assess whether an individual felt stressed, researchers asked questions about whether the individuals felt loved and supported by friends and family. For those who did not feel supported, the five-year death rate was 50 percent. Among those who had a supportive and loving family, the five-year death rate was just 15 percent.

Now that we have some idea of the negative impact stress has on our bodies, how do we identify if we are stressed, what is stressing us out, and what do we do about it?

In an attempt to quantify stress, psychiatrists Thomas Holmes and Richard Rahe developed the *Holmes-Rahe Social Readjustment Rating Scale* in 1967. It assigns points to major life events and scores the risk for developing stress related illnesses. At the top of the list were death of a spouse, divorce, death of another close family member, serious illness, jail term, being fired from a job, and a new marriage. It is important to note that while the events do carry a significant amount of stress, the way we respond to the events (often times influenced by past experiences) also plays a significant role.

Table 4: Holmes-Rahe Social Readjustment Rating Scale

Event	Value	Event	Value
Death of spouse	100	Son or daughter leaving home	29
Divorce	73	Trouble with in-laws	29
Marital separation	65	Outstanding personal achievement	28
Jail term	63	Spouse begins or ceases working	26
Death of close family member	63	Starting or finishing school	26
Personal injury or illness	53	Change in living conditions	25
Marriage	50	Revision of personal habits	24
Fired from job	47	Trouble with boss	23
Marital reconciliation	45	Change in work hours, conditions	20
Retirement	45	Change in residence	20
Change in family member's health	44	Change in schools	20
Pregnancy	40	Change in recreational habits	19
Sexual difficulties	39	Change in church activities	19
Addition to family	39	Change in social activities	18
Business readjustment	39	Mortgage or loan under $10, 000	17
Change in financial status	38	Change in sleeping habits	15
Death of close friend	37	Change in number of family gatherings	15
Career change	36	Change in eating habits	15
Change in number of marital arguments	35	Vacation	13
Mortgage or loan over $10,000	31	Christmas season	12
Foreclosure of mortgage or loan	30	Minor violation of the law	11
Change in work responsibilities	29		

How you respond to a stressful situation can go long way to help reduce risk of chronic disorders. In fact, the way you view the problems in life can actually be just as important as the events themselves. It is important that you seek professional help if you are feeling overwhelmed or have any concerns about your mental and/or physical health. Below are some examples of major life events and some possible coping strategies.

1. **Moving to a New City**
   In this economy, getting a job may require you and your family to move. Whether you're headed across the country or across town, moving can be one of life's biggest stressors. There is comfort in the "same old, same old," and most of us do not like change. Change shakes us up in more ways than one and forces us out of our comfort zone.

   Why not looking at moving to a new town as a fresh start? Ask yourself what positive changes you would like to make in your new life. You may want to join a new gym or start each day by walking around your new neighborhood with your dog. Use the move as an opportunity to start fresh and set new goals for yourself.

   Staying in touch with old contacts, family and friends is easy using today's technology. Those folks will appreciate being included in your new life as well.

   No matter how much you may love your new home or job, it is normal to mourn the old life you left behind. Elisabeth Kübler Ross, M.D. identified the five stages of grief in her book, *On Death and Dying,* published in 1969. They are:

   - Anger

- Denial
- Bargaining
- Depression
- Acceptance

Acknowledge each stage of the grieving process and allow yourself the time to process each one. It is not good to stop the grieving process, so let it happen. Consider professional help to work through your feelings during this difficult time. If you move for your job, the company may offer counseling through an employee assistance program (EAP).

2. Stress of Losing Your Job

In the midst of the high national unemployment rate, millions of people feel stressed because they are struggling to keep their job or finding a new one if they have been laid off. Record numbers of Americans are struggling every day trying to pay rent and feed their families in this unstable economy. Even as early as 2001, unemployment, debt and homelessness advanced on the list of top 10 stressful life events that led to physical and mental illness, as measured by the Holmes-Rahe Life Stress Inventory.

Grieving the loss of a job involves taking time to acknowledge the pain and anger so that negative emotions are not bottled deep inside. It's important to continue self-care by exercising, eating right and staying healthy so that you meet new job opportunities in the best frame of mind. Starting or keeping up an exercise routine activates feel-good hormones, gets you out of the house and provides structure (something that can fall apart after a job loss). Plus, healthy eating and exercise give your self-esteem a boost at a very vulnerable time and prepares your body to cope with stress and anxiety.

Avoid self-medicating with junk food. Focus on foods like fruits, vegetables, whole grains, and lean protein sources, such as chicken and fish. Drink plenty of water to stay hydrated and energized.

Remember to keep your attitude in the right place– otherwise, you could set yourself up for failure and despair. Try to keep fear out of the equation, and adopt an attitude of abundance. A hopeful mindset will keep you energized and inspire you to take action and realize your dreams. Learn from your job loss by asking yourself, "What could I have done differently?" Take what you have learned and apply it to your new job.

Consider turning to others for help. Family and friends may be willing to help if they are aware of your situation. Find out about federal, state and municipal unemployment support programs. Community organizations, like your church or college alma mater, may have additional resources available to you.

3. Breakup or Divorce

Even if the decision to breakup is a good one, the end of a partnership and shared history with another person is still painful. Feeling overwhelmed by feelings of regret, failure and shame are a normal part of the process. This kind of stress is difficult to navigate alone because your emotions can cloud your thinking and actions.

Focus on the good things that will come from the breakup, even though you may feel sad, angry and upset. It might be the right time to take a new class, make a career change, or relocate to a new city and make a fresh start.

Lean on close friends and family who will offer support and give you a hug when you need one. Your support system can keep you thinking rationally, give you a shoulder to cry on, or provide a sounding board for new ideas. You may also wish to seek professional help a qualified mental health therapist or find comfort in your spiritual or religious practices.

4. Health Diagnosis
Take the time to learn all you can about any unexpected health diagnosis. Seek out the experts in and gather information about treatment options and care. Do something healthy for yourself every day, such as exercise, to lower your stress levels. Create a lifestyle plan. Again, call on friends, family and community resources for support.

5. Empty Nest Syndrome
No matter how proud you are when your children head off to college, you are likely to feel a sense of emptiness and may need to fight the urge to call them every day. For women, it can be especially tough to step back in the role as a mother that required a great deal of dedication over many years. Again, recognizing the five stages of grief and allowing yourself experience the process, while caring for your emotional and physical self, are crucial steps. Just like a move to a new home or town, the empty nest syndrome can be approached with a sense of exploration and adventure. Embrace new hobbies and interests, volunteer, go back to work, or decide to pursue an advanced degree. Make a plan and take daily steps to create a new future.

Now I know that it is not possible to mention every potential stressor, especially since the stress response is based in part by our individual response to the event. What creates a stress response in one person may not create the same response in another. So here is my advice to cope when feeling overwhelmed: keep it **F.F.R.E.S.H:**

F: Find and fix any underlying conditions. Identify the source of the stress and create a plan of action. Now that may mean instituting stress management techniques such as meditation, breathing exercises, yoga or other activities that are soothing to the body, like a lavender bath. It may also include seeking professional help to sort through emotions, patterns and identify any underlying health issues.

F: Food is medicine. Start making healthy food choices. The fatigue and fogginess that can accompany stress only gets worse if poor nutrition is added. Keep in mind that poor nutrition is also a stressor. Poor food choices can contribute to weight gain and inflammation in the body.

R: Relationships are important. They can be nourishing or they can be toxic. People who feel connected and supported tend to live longer, healthier lives. Cultivate the relationships that nourish you and identify the ones that are toxic.

E: Exercise. It is one of the best stress management tools available to us. It can be as simple as taking a walk around the block or practicing yoga. Daily exercise offers benefits like an improved mood; a decreased risk of chronic disorders, like osteoporosis and diabetes; and helps us maintain a healthy weight.

S: Sleep. Your body needs time to rejuvenate and your mind needs time to process and put the events of the day into prospective. Without adequate sleep your ability to focus and problem solve becomes significantly compromised.

H: Happiness. To paraphrase my favorite quote: happiness stems from the serenity to accept the things you cannot change, the strength to change the things you can, and the wisdom to know the difference.

**

UPDATE:

Kate had no major upheavals in her life, but she had failed to prioritize and nurture her mental health and well-being for years. Her life felt overwhelming and the demands of her job and family left her feeling that she had little time to take care of herself. By not taking care herself mentally and physically, Kate felt tired, foggy and even a little resentful of the people and situations she felt were taking advantage of her time. Feeling guilty that she wasn't able to prioritize and do it all, Kate compensated by taking on even more projects and responsibilities.

During her course of treatment, Kate came to the realization that she needed to change the way she perceived self-care. I reminded her that there is no system designed to continuously perform without replenishing its resources—not cars, not Mother Nature and certainly not humans. Giving our body, mind and spirit what they need to flourish allows us to be present for others in a positive way. By viewing self-care as an essential part of her health, Kate was able to plan time into her daily calendar for her own stress management and lifestyle adjustments.

Simple STEP 6
Let Your Brain Work For You And
Keep It Young

Your brain is wonderfully complex. It uses very powerful chemicals, known as neurotransmitters, to communicate. These neurotransmitters can help control your appetite as well as modulate your moods. Certain emotions and stressors in life affect the chemical balance in the brain. What may appear to be a lack of willpower could potentially be an unbalanced level of neurotransmitters. You can learn to give your brain the ability to soothe your emotions, to relieve stress, and indulge in pleasure and balance in more effective and satisfying ways.

Brain Biology and Cravings
Do you often feel a powerful drive to overeat when stressed or to eat foods that you know aren't good for you? Do you feel guilty about your inability to control these urges and feel you are developing self-destructive habits? Do you ever wonder what causes these compelling urges? Wouldn't it be nice to know that there might be a biological reason behind what you feel and that you're not just going crazy? Let's explore the science behind what makes you susceptible to crave certain unhealthy foods and eventually cave into the strong desire to overeat.

More than 100,000 chemical reactions take place in the brain every second. Communication between the brain and nerve cells is the basis behind everything you think, feel and do. The brain uses neurotransmitters as messengers that signal nerves throughout the body, regulating the way you feel throughout the day; some cause increased alertness, while others cause more calming effects. The neurotransmitters that keep us alert are referred to as excitatory; those that bring calmness are referred to as inhibitory. It is the balance between these two components that can make us feel anxious (too much excitatory or too little calming) or fatigued (too little excitatory or too much inhibitory). Balance helps us to stay alert during the day, sleep well at night, enjoy our lives, and maintain a balanced weight.

You might not realize that what you eat can affect the formation of these neurotransmitters and play a significant effect on your mood, appetite and cravings. Before discussing the specific neurotransmitters that directly affect your appetite and moods, let's discuss the relationship between behavior and balance in the brain.

Your brain is constantly trying to achieve balance. This also applies to your mood. For instance, if you're overly stressed, the brain needs to achieve balance by calling for an action that will release neurotransmitters that bring more calmness and relaxation to the body. The brain quickly learns to associate things that we do with pleasure or bringing about a sense of calmness. Once associations are formed, like Pavlov's dogs, our behavior may become a conditioned response or a knee-jerk reaction, to do the quickest, easiest and most well-conditioned action that will help release neurotransmitters. Eating is usually the easiest and quickest solution. Plus, the smell, taste and appearance of food can excite the chemicals within the brain that lead to intense pleasure, stress release, and emotional satisfaction. Whatever our brain associates with quick, instantaneous gratification and pleasure is what we will do repeatedly. It's what we've been conditioned to do.

In the next section, let's take a deeper look at how neurotransmitters in the brain work so that we can discover alternatives to unwanted habitual cycles.

Serotonin, Endorphins and Dopamine: Appetite and Mood Regulators

Serotonin
Serotonin is probably the most heavily researched neurotransmitter and is a very powerful mood enhancer and appetite regulator. When released, it brings about feelings of calmness, happiness, serenity and satisfaction. Sufficient amounts of circulating serotonin also signal feelings of fullness and reduced appetite. Low levels of serotonin are linked to depression and increased appetite. Many anti-depressants work by increasing availability of circulating serotonin in the brain.

Dietary Influences on Serotonin
It's probably no coincidence that when you're stressed or feeling blue you might turn to sweets, baked goods, desserts, and other sugary carbohydrates to calm down. Carbohydrate rich foods raise brain concentrations of an amino acid called tryptophan, which is the building block for serotonin. Eating carbohydrates enhances the production of serotonin in the brain and makes us feel relaxed. Likewise, a high protein diet can suppress formation of serotonin levels, which might decrease feelings of calmness and relaxation, but can enhance mental alertness.

However, eating sugary carbohydrates, instead of complex carbohydrates, can actually have a rebound effect on your mood. You might feel good immediately after eating these sugary carbs because they lead to an instant high and a quick energy boost. But, shortly afterwards, your blood sugar and energy levels drop significantly, which can actually cause a rebound depression, or "sugar low." This can, in turn, stimulate more sugary carbohydrate cravings to get back to the initial "sugar high." Plus, eating does not really combat stress in a long-term or effective way as overeating generally leads to increased feelings of guilt.

Endorphins

Endorphins are very powerful natural opiates in the brain that produce feelings of intense pleasure. They can also reduce and relieve pain. You might have heard of the term "runner's high" that refers to the release of feel-good endorphins after a long run or exercise session.

Dietary Influences on Endorphins

Some research postulates that sugar/fat combinations can enhance the production of endorphins. You might crave foods, such as chocolate, precisely because of its high fat/high sugar content. Chocolate contains phenylethylamine (PEA), an endorphin-releasing substance. In fact, any food with a high sugar and fat content such as doughnuts, baked goods, and ice cream can increase endorphin and serotonin levels. That's quite an irresistible combination, especially when you feel blue or stressed and need a quick "high" or mood lift.

Dopamine

Dopamine is a neurotransmitter that can increase mental alertness and awareness. Dopamine is also one of major neurotransmitters involved in the "reward" center of the brain. Studies suggest that this reward center and dopamine are implicated in addictive behavior. Food is one way to stimulate the release of dopamine in the brain. In recent studies, obese individuals were found to have lower dopamine activity in the reward center of the brain. One theory is that there is a lower dopamine activity rate in the brain of obese individuals, so more food is consumed in an attempt to stimulate that pleasure reward center. Research continues to be done to delineate the role of this important neurotransmitter in overeating and other addictive behavior.

Another important role of dopamine is to help regulate procedural learning and movement in the body. In diseases such as Parkinson's where dopamine concentration is reduced in the brain, patients report issues with learning and movement disorders. Studies show that dopamine may also play a role in regulating our circadian rhythm (our wake and sleep cycle) by increasing our clock protein, PER2.

Brain-derived Neurotrophic Factor
Brain-derived neurotrophic factor (BDNF) is a substance within the brain that has been shown to protect brain cells and help them survive under stressful conditions. These cells are also found in other parts of the body, such as the heart. Studies suggest that positive thoughts reinforce optimal production of this substance, and circumstances perceived as negative or stressful induce the release of glutamate, a substance that is toxic in high amounts and can lead to the death of numerous brain cells.

As we get older, our brains produce more glutamate in response to stress—five times higher than when we are younger, according to some studies. Furthermore, as we age the brain becomes slower to clear this toxic substance away. Together, this adds up to prolonged toxic exposure and increased cell death. Since glutamate has an affinity for the memory cells, a buildup could manifest as issues with short-term memory recollection and other symptoms.

The results of some animal studies show that the brain's ability to produce and modulate BDNF in response to stressful situations can be significantly compromised if the animal suffers significant stress in infancy, such as parental separation. It may also not surprise us to learn that the longer the distressing episode lasts, the less protection is offered by BDNF. As with most health crises, the very old and the very young appear to be most susceptible.

Cravings, Overeating & Emotions - The Brain Chemistry Connection

There are things that occur every day that can cause significant changes and shifts in the brain chemicals. As the brain seeks balance when negative emotions and stressors surface, it immediately looks for pleasure and balance from previous responses to foods. Often, we are not aware of our emotions or stressors, nor that we are overeating in response to these emotions, until we make a habit of "becoming in tune with" or paying attention to how we really feel.

Some common factors can affect your brain chemistry and your cravings. Stress, fear, anger, and anxiety can induce a series of chemical reactions in the body that prompt cravings, cause weight gain or make it difficult to lose weight. Prolonged stress can lower serotonin levels, increase cortisol levels and increase insulin levels. All of these changes can increase cravings (especially for sweets), cause mood swings, and increase the risk for chronic lifestyle illness such as Type 2 diabetes and heart disease. Stress can also increase the production of a neurotransmitter called neuropeptide Y, which can significantly increase carbohydrate cravings and has been shown to increase abdominal fat. Neuropeptide Y is secreted by the part of the brain called the hypothalamus.

So what foods can you choose when you're feeling stressed? Let's explore some food options that can help us achieve a balanced brain in a healthy way.

Foods that Support Neurotransmitter Health

Protein is broken down into its amino acid components during digestion. The amino acid tyrosine is used to increase the production of dopamine, norepinephrine, and epinephrine in the brain. These neurotransmitters have the ability to increase our alertness and boost energy levels. Eating foods high in protein—such as fish, meat and eggs—will increase the amount of tyrosine available and may provide a slight mental boost. Carbohydrate foods that also contain significant amounts of protein, such as legumes, cheese, milk or tofu may also produce the same effect.

Carbohydrates trigger the release of insulin into the blood stream. Insulin clears all the amino acids (except tryptophan) from the bloodstream. Tryptophan is normally crowded out by other amino acids in an attempt to cross the blood-brain barrier. However, when its competitors are out of the way, tryptophan is able to enter the brain and is converted to serotonin, a neurotransmitter that has the effect of reducing pain, decreasing appetite, producing a sense of calm, and (with large quantities) inducing sleep.

Despite its bad rap, caffeine in moderation is beneficial to the body. Long-term epidemiological evidence supports the effectiveness of a cup or two of coffee a daily to help reduce risk of depression. Consuming larger quantities can have counterproductive effects in some people.

Folic acid also is an important remedy to fight depression. Folic acid deficiencies have been linked to depression in clinical studies because they cause serotonin levels in the brain to decrease. Psychiatric patients with depression have much higher rates of folic acid deficiency than the public population. As little as 200 micrograms per day is enough to relieve depression, an amount easily obtained from a cup of cooked spinach, a whole orange, or a glass of fresh-squeezed orange juice.

Individuals suffering from a lack of selenium have been shown to be more anxious, irritable, hostile, and depressed than those with normal levels. Correcting deficiencies normalizes moods, but ingesting a higher amount does not further elevate moods and can be harmful. Though it seems to have some neural function, selenium's precise mode of action is unknown. Selenium rich foods include Brazil nuts, sunflower seeds, whole grain cereals, tuna, and swordfish.

In the fervor to avoid cholesterol, many people become deficient in choline, a B-complex vitamin that is concentrated in high-cholesterol foods, such as eggs and liver. A lack of choline can cause impairment of memory and concentration. Choline is a precursor to the brain neurotransmitter, acetylcholine, which is linked to memory loss. People on certain medications that block acetylcholine often flunk memory tests, and low levels of acetylcholine have been linked to Alzheimer's disease and poor memory.

Non-Emotional Factors Related to Depressed Serotonin Levels

These factors are unrelated to stress, but can also cause a drop in serotonin levels.

1. PMS is a series of symptoms, such as irritability, anxiety and bloating, that occurs shortly after mid-cycle ovulation and resolves usually at the onset of the

menstrual cycle. Studies suggest that serotonin may play a role in PMS. It seems that serotonin levels tend to fall after ovulation and could potentially contribute to the symptomology. There might actually be a true biological reason behind those chocolate cravings during a certain time of the month!

2. Seasonal Affective Disorder (SAD) is the amount of natural sunlight you are exposed to each day affects serotonin levels. Those who live in areas (especially people living in Northern climates that experience fewer daylight hours during the winter months than Southern regions) often report increased feelings of depression and increased cravings for carbohydrates.

3. Excessive protein in the diet can suppress serotonin levels. Many people who consume high protein diets report a decreased ability to feel calm and relaxed and an increased craving for carbohydrates.

It's important to recognize when we experience periods of difficult emotions and stress. Many of us will go through the following cycle:

- Stress, emotional swings
- Depressed serotonin levels
- Brain seeks balance (wants to be calm)
- Eat high carbohydrate or high carbohydrate/high fat foods
- Raise endorphins and serotonin
- Feel sedated, relaxed and even "high"
- Sugary foods lead to only a quick, temporary increase in energy
- Blood sugar levels drop, energy drops, "sugar low" feelings set in
- More cravings for carbohydrates and fats to make you feel calm and relaxed again

Your brain also quickly learns this pattern. You have trained it to realize that when you have any myriad feelings, like stress, depression, or anger, eating certain foods will help "numb out" those feelings by releasing powerful mood-altering neurotransmitters. Your brain will continue to seek stress and emotional relief from the cycle until you learn to break it.

Conquer your emotions and stress effectively without overeating

Stress, feeling blue, fear, and guilt are a normal part of life. Chances are, we can't fully rid ourselves of these unpleasant feelings, but we can learn to deal with them more effectively. Our objective reasoning tells us that eating unhealthy foods isn't resolving our stress or emotional problems. But that thinking isn't very helpful when our brain is screaming, "Eat, eat, I want to be calm."

Just as you trained your brain that eating certain foods can lead to greater feelings of calm and relaxation (albeit temporarily), you can train it to seek other sources of pleasure that also increase mood-enhancing neurotransmitters. Unlike overeating, these alternative sources of pleasure will offer an additional benefit of a healthier lifestyle.

Some people can simply recognize the problem and decide not to eat and "ride out the urge." But, for many, that is only a temporary and not an effective long-term solution. Your brain will continually prompt you to find something to give it balance and pleasure when facing stressful and emotional situations. It is difficult to consistently ignore these urges. What you can do is replace one pleasure (eating) with another pleasure (meditation, exercise, etc.) to effectively satisfy your urges.

It can take some time, but eventually, you might begin to crave a long run or vigorous workout to boost your endorphins instead of indulging in a piece of chocolate cake. It's all a matter of retraining your brain. Generally speaking, anything that brings you personal pleasure, inspiration, or a sense of well-being without harming your health is what you should act on when food cravings and the drive to overeat takes over.

Modify Eating Habits

Some people report decreased cravings when they modify their diet. You can try some of these techniques and see if any work for you:

- Eat breakfast to improve performance, and mood to start your day off right. Eating breakfast helps avoid overeating at lunch or dinner.
- Eat smaller snacks throughout the day and only eat when you are physically hungry.
- Become familiar with your body's signals. Don't eat because it's mealtime. Eat when you're hungry and stop when you're satisfied, not stuffed.
- Eat a balance of high protein and high carbohydrate foods at meals to keep blood sugar levels normalized.
- Satisfy your carbohydrate cravings with complex carbohydrates like whole wheat bread, low fat crackers, low fat popcorn, whole grain cereals, beans, whole grain pastas, and brown rice. Your body absorbs complex carbohydrates slower than sugars so you won't feel a rise and fall in sugar levels, causing mood swings.
- Eat more high fiber foods to feel full longer and minimize hunger.
- Eat a balanced diet. Do not significantly restrict fat or carbohydrates or go on a starvation diet. Your body requires all of the nutrients in a balanced diet to function properly.

- Limit or avoid alcohol since it acts as a depressant.

The following steps may be helpful to you when your brain seeks pleasure and stress relief.

1. **Exercise**. Yet another reason to do it. It increases endorphin levels and relieves stress. You'll feel inspired and good about yourself, and you'll naturally decrease your food cravings.
2. **Get a massage**. It may help relieve anxiety, depression and alleviate sleep problems.
3. **Get inspired.** Seek out people and things that inspire you.
4. **Meditate**. Repeat a positive word, phrase or prayer. It minimizes distracting, negative thoughts and relieves stress.
5. **Use guided imagery**. Think about your favorite place for 10-15 minutes with your eyes closed. It might be the mountains, the beach, or other favorite spot. Imagine everything you're seeing, hearing, smelling, and feeling.
6. **Listen to relaxing music**. Studies have shown that listening to relaxing music (like jazz or classical) decreases the production of a substance called cortisol that can lead to carbohydrate cravings. Music can also increase relaxation, relieve stress, and provide more clarity and vigor.
7. **Indulge in aromatherapy**. Oils of eucalyptus, lavender, and chamomile added to a warm bath can instantly invigorate the senses and relax tired muscles.
8. **Laugh**. See a comedy show, or engage in activities that bring humor to your life. Seek ways to have more positive emotions in your life. Finding the positive always overrides the negative.

9. **Get a pet and love it**. Studies show that pets add unconditional love to our lives and can reduce blood pressure and stress.
10. **Journal** your feelings or talk to someone you can trust.
11. **Plan a fun group activity** with family or friends that you enjoy.
12. **Keep learning:** Learning new skills and information helps to keep the brain young.
13. Go through **old photo albums** and scrapbooks. Recall happy times and make plans for new ventures.
14. **Treat yourself** to a gift, like a book, a magazine, a new dress, or a manicure.
15. **Consider volunteering** for a charity or organization that has significance for you. Studies suggest that people who volunteer have stronger social networks and a more positive attitude.

Reach Out and Touch Someone

As a society, we should find more ways for people, especially the elderly, to stay involved and active. At any age, we need to begin to think beyond the boundaries of the stairmaster or treadmill.

Physical fitness is very important, but social engagement is just as critical to longevity. Find something you really enjoy doing that involves group interaction, whether it's playing cards, power walking in the mall, or volunteering with your church or local charity. Social engagement adds a sense of purpose to a person's life and years to your health in the process.

Social Interaction and Immunity

People who have the strong support of friends or spouses typically feel a greater sense of self-esteem and take better care of themselves by adopting a healthy lifestyle. A strong social network may also help reduce stress and there is evidence that indicates an increased psychological and physical well-being. A study performed at Ohio State University showed people who are lonely or socially isolated show signs of a suppressed immune system. Boosting one's immune system is an essential part of warding off illness and staying healthy. In a study published in *Psychosomatic Medicine,* researchers found that patients who scored above the median level on loneliness tests had significantly fewer active natural killer cells – cells that attack germs.

The techniques mentioned are not intended to address serious emotional issues that require professional help and counseling. If you feel that you have a problem with a binge eating disorder, like anorexia or bulimia, seek help immediately from your physician, psychologist or mental health counselor.

**

UPDATE:

Kate's eating and lifestyle patterns had depleted her serotonin levels. She craved sweets constantly as her body attempted to replenish the levels of this neurotransmitter. Kate routinely ate sweets that would trigger the release of high amounts of insulin and then her blood sugar levels would drop precipitously an hour later. Then a "fight or flight" response was created by the body, dramatically increasing cortisol and adrenaline levels that left Kate hungry, shaky and anxious. Persistently elevated cortisol and adrenaline levels could eventually contribute towards high blood pressure, an increased risk for Type 2 diabetes and make it difficult to lose weight. The vicious cycle was repeatedly daily and hard to break.

We discussed other healthier steps for Kate to restore her sense of calm instead of reaching for a cookie or other sugary foods. We also wanted to keep Kate's brain healthy so we included Omega-3's into her daily eating plan. Study published in the *Alzheimer & Dementia Journal* showed that 900mg of DHA (an important component of omega-3 essential fatty acid) improved memory and learning with aging. We created a menu plan with lean protein combined with green leafy vegetables and some complex carbohydrates to help maximize her usage of the amino acid tryptophan. Green leafy vegetables are an excellent source of folic acid, which promotes a sense of emotional well-being.

Kate realized that other interventions might be needed if her symptoms did not improve significantly with these lifestyle changes. She understood but expressed a strong desire to follow through with the changes first before using other modalities.

Simple STEP 7
Anti-Aging and Supplements

What is aging and why do we age? These eternal questions have created a billion dollar a year cosmetic industry to make us feel and look younger. We know aging can have internal and external manifestations. For example, internal aging can manifest as an accelerated rate of heart disease, or the hardening of blood vessels that leads to high blood pressure. The signs of external aging are far more visible. Poor muscle tone, a significant increase in abdominal fat, sagging, loose or prematurely aging skin that loses its youthful glow, leaving a dull, lifeless complexion are some noticeable changes. Are all of these changes inevitable? Why are some 70-year-olds jumping out of planes, competing in body building competitions and running marathons, while some 50-year-olds can't seem to walk a flight of stairs without getting winded?

While some products claim to turn back the hands of time, can they really do it? Here's a look at the facts. First, it is widely accepted that as we age, many of our body's functions slow down and become less efficient. We lose muscle mass at the rate of 1 percent a year after the age of 30. As we enter perimenopause (or andropause, for men), signaling the fall of our youthful sex hormones, such as estrogen and testosterone, we may start gaining weight and become more tired, indicating an imbalance in our other hormones such as insulin, thyroid hormone and cortisol.

While no one has discovered the magic bullet (contrary to the commercials that bombard us daily) that will completely halt the aging process, current research has revealed opportunities to slow down the process. To understand how these interventions could possibly work, let us consider some of the hypotheses behind the science of aging.

Inflammation

One main theory targets chronic inflammation, a condition believed to play a significant role in developing cardiovascular disease, diabetes, allergies, cancer and other long-term, debilitating illnesses. When there is injury to tissues, our immune system generates an inflammatory response, sending out macrophages (white blood cells) to ingest foreign particles and infectious microorganisms in an attempt to clear out and repair the damage. The role of the initial acute inflammatory stage is to defend the body from infections, help it heal and return it to natural balance. If an infectious agent triggers this response in our body, we are on way to restored health.

However, infections aren't the only things that can trigger an immune response. Other conditions such as elevated cholesterol levels or an increase in the fatty molecules along the walls of the arteries that supply blood to heart can also trigger inflammation. Immune cells enter, and the inflammatory response generated can lead to the breaking apart of the fatty lesions. This triggers the clotting mechanism—creating blood clots that can break off and block arteries, causing a heart attack.

Unfortunately, the inflammatory process also produces damaging chemicals known as cytokines and free radicals. Cytokines are messengers that recruit more immune cells and other responders to help in the battle. Free radicals, or reactive oxygen species, help destroy other invaders, but can also damage normal tissue.

Studies have indeed linked inflammation to Alzheimer's disease, heart disease, osteoporosis, sarcopenia (muscle loss), arthritis, and several other chronic disorders. Obesity can increase inflammation because fat cells have the ability to initiate the inflammatory cascade. Studies show that people within a normal weight range with an elevated percentage of body fat (i.e., greater than 30 percent for women) are at an increased risk for hypertension, dyslipidemia (abnormal levels of fats and cholesterol in the blood), and cardiovascular disease.

Chronic inflammation can be a low-grade, festering process that can linger for years. Triggers can range from oxidized, damaged cholesterol to common bacteria or viruses that most of us have been exposed to at some point in our lives.

Free Radical/Oxidation Theory
Another theory of aging involves oxidation. Oxidation is a process when the cells cycle on a daily basis to produce energy. During this process, unstable elements known as free radicals are produced. The body has a mechanism in place to neutralize these molecules; however, antioxidants, such as vitamin C, can significantly modify this process. Insufficient amounts of antioxidants or excessive production of free radicals can lead to excessive cellular damage, accelerating the aging process and contributing to chronic illness. Damage from these elements can activate the immune system, and generate additional free radicals, creating a cycle that can be hard to break.

Acceleration of heart disease, chronic fatigue, and the aging of the skin have all been linked to this theory. It is also believed factors such as smoking, poor diet, or a stressful home or work environment can increase the rate of oxidation, promoting faster aging and chronic illness.

Hormonal Theory

Evidence is mounting that the decline in steroid hormone levels as we age is one of the leading causes in the decline of our physical and mental function. Steroid hormones are derived from the cholesterol molecule. Through several complex chemical reactions, cholesterol is converted into our sex hormones: estrogen, testosterone and progesterone.

Our hormonal levels may start declining as early as in our thirties. For women, the symptoms become more noticeable at the early stages of menopause, known as perimenopause. Menopause is defined as the absence of menstrual periods for 12 consecutive months with no other identifiable biological cause. Studies suggest that the decline of our hormones can be accompanied by a series of conditions that compromise not only our quality of life, but also our health.

It is estimated that during menopause, 20 percent of women suffer from depression and up to 50 percent of women suffer from insomnia. Men in andropause show an increased risk of depression, insomnia and health issues such as osteoporosis and cardiovascular dysfunction. Physicians also know that depression and insomnia can increase the risk for weight gain, cardiovascular disease and insulin resistance. Let's take a closer look at each of the major players in this hormonal game.

Testosterone

Testosterone is the major sex hormone in men, but is also present in lower quantities in women. Dwindling levels of testosterone can cause a decrease in virility and strength in both men and women. Low levels have also been associated with depression, osteoporosis and low recovery levels in men with congestive heart failure. One study suggests that depression and low testosterone levels were both associated with an increased risk of poor outcomes in heart failure patients. In men, low testosterone levels have also been associated with an increased risk of insomnia.

There is a circadian rhythm to the release of testosterone in men. In younger men, there is an early morning rise in the levels of testosterone. These high-peak morning levels of testosterone are the first to be affected as men age. Therefore, evaluations for testosterone deficiencies should be performed in the morning because late day results may not accurately represent the body's lowest levels.

Testosterone replacement therapy is becoming more widely accepted as a treatment option to enhance the male sense of well-being. Therapy can improve sleep quality and body composition (i.e., the ratio of fat to muscle) and reduce symptoms of depression and low libido. It also seems to protect against mortality from congestive heart failure. There appears to be no link between testosterone replacement therapy and prostate cancer. However, it is prudent for physicians to monitor the prostate regularly with digital rectal exams and blood tests for prostate-specific antigen levels.

Recent studies suggest that testosterone may offer some benefit to women as well. It seems to contribute to the maintenance of good bone density in older women. Some studies suggest it may counteract the proliferative effects of estrogen and progesterone on breast cells. However, whether this equates to a reduced risk of breast cancer has yet to be determined.

Estrogen

Estrogen is one of the major reproductive hormones in women and is present in lower concentrations in men.

As estrogen levels decline in women, some notable changes take place. The skin and hair become drier and thinner. Collagen loss increases and the appearance of fine lines and wrinkles on the face and hands become more definitive. Women often begin experiencing insomnia, irritability, anxiety, panic attacks, depression, elevated blood pressure, as well as weight gain or the redistribution of weight. Risks for osteoporosis and heart disease also increase.

A boost of estrogen seems to play a significant role in preventing the skin from aging by increasing the body's production of collagen, which supports the skin's barrier function by producing moisture-containing molecules that help maintain the skin's elasticity, suppleness, strength and thickness. In addition to the positive effects on the skin, healthy estrogen levels contribute to the maintenance of bone and muscle mass, increase the metabolic rate and decrease the risk of heart disease among women by as much as 50 percent. Estrogen supports a healthy blood pressure and improves the quality of one's sleep and moods.

Studies suggest that estrogen replacement therapy (ERT) may have a triphasic effect on the cardiovascular system, offering both benefits and risks at differing times over the course of treatment. If ERT is initiated at the onset of menopause, then estrogen replacement seems to reduce one's risk of cardiovascular disease by reducing plaque formation. However, if therapy is delayed until years after menopause, when plaque has already formed, it can increase the risk that the plaque will rupture, leading to a heart attack. Interestingly, estrogen therapy may offer an additional benefit by improving the cholesterol ratio (i.e., decreasing LDL and increasing HDL) in later years.

Research indicates that estrogen's effects on our moods are mediated through the hormone's ability to amplify the effects of serotonin and endorphins in the brain. Both serotonin and endorphins help improve our feelings of comfort and promote a positive mood. Estrogen also has the important effect of enhancing the action and production of the memory neurotransmitter, acetylcholine.

Of course, estrogen therapy is not the solution for every woman and should be completely evaluated by a physician after weighing a patient's personal medical history and known risk factors.

Progesterone
Progesterone is a reproductive hormone that works in concert with estrogen to regulate the menstrual cycle, prepare the body for pregnancy, and support it during gestation. Progesterone is produced primarily by the ovaries and in small amounts by the adrenal glands. The hormone is produced after ovulation (release of egg by the ovary). During pregnancy, the placenta can also produce progesterone. Progesterone in the body can be converted into testosterone and corticosteroids (used in the stress response).

Aside from its actions in our reproductive cycle, progesterone has been shown in laboratory studies to increase the synthesis of osteoblasts (the cells responsible for rebuilding bone tissue). When combined with estrogen, the effects were even more pronounced. The results suggest that progesterone could be helpful in preventing or improving osteoporosis. Although anecdotal reports and individual case studies support progesterone's independent role in increasing bone density, currently there is not enough major clinical research to support using progesterone alone for that purpose. However, in combination with estrogen therapy, the results have been promising.

When it comes to improving sleep patterns and reducing anxiety, progesterone's primary role has received stronger validation. Chronic, persistent insomnia and anxiety can cause weight gain and increase the risks of inflammation and insulin resistance—all contributing to the body's aging. Progesterone and its derivative allopregnanolone have been shown to bind to receptors in the brain and induce a relaxation response similar to benzodiazepines (e.g. Valium). Sleep studies show that it can improve quality of sleep for patients who suffer with sleep disturbances. Several studies demonstrate that women require less anesthetic during the phase of their menstrual cycles where progesterone production is the highest, further demonstrating progesterone's relaxation effects. Animal studies on male rats showed a similar response to anesthesia when progesterone was administered.

Progesterone in larger amounts can exacerbate depression symptoms. Because progesterone levels tend to be low among menopausal women, this is usually not a problem. However, if replacement therapy is instituted, progesterone levels and patient response need to be carefully monitored by a qualified medical professional for any changes in mental behavior.

Cortisol

Cholesterol is also the basic component of the stress hormones cortisol and DHEA. In the body, replenishing the stress response hormones takes precedence over replenishing sex hormones—survival trumps reproduction and libido. Since both our sex hormones and stress hormones are built from the same raw materials, excessive stress can lead to an early decline in our sex hormones, and possibly contribute to early onset of menopause in women, or andropause in men.

Research strongly correlates reciprocal increases in stress and cholesterol. An overly simplified explanation is that the body's production of cholesterol rises to meet the demand for cortisol and DHEA required to combat increased stress levels. One study noted that stress caused the blood to clot much faster. A combination of higher cholesterol and higher rate of blood clotting could be a recipe for premature heart disease and stroke. In fact, one elegant study published in the *European Heart Journal* in 2008 followed 10,000 civil servants over a 12-year period to assess the effects of work stress on heart disease. The findings indicate that the risk of heart disease among the test subjects that suffered from prolonged work stress increased by 68 percent. These individuals showed higher than normal cortisol levels throughout the day, as compared to their counterparts. The study's authors noted that the poor lifestyle habits developed in response to the stress created an additional risk.

As we get older, our bodies are slower to adapt to stress. Our brain cells become more susceptible to the effects of stress hormones. Cortisol can damage the area in the brain that is responsible for short-term memory, thus contributing to forgetfulness often referred to as "brain fog." These effects can be compounded by the decline in the production of sex hormones. For example, estrogen supports the production and action of acetylcholine, known as the memory neurotransmitter. The bottom line is that stress can increase our cortisol levels and decrease our estrogen and testosterone levels, thereby making brain cells more susceptible to injury.

Prolonged stress along with a corresponding increase in cortisol production can lead to deficiencies in vitamins B6,

B12, and folate. These vitamins play a critical role in maintaining a healthy nervous system, mood and energy level, as well as the production of healthy blood cells. For example, vitamin B6 plays an important part in production of the neurotransmitter serotonin that helps boost our moods, relieve our anxiety, and improve our sleep quality.

An imbalance in cortisol levels can also contribute to blood sugar levels measuring too high or too low. If cortisol is not well regulated, blood pressure, immunity, energy and mood can become compromised.

Thyroid hormones

Thyroid hormones can diminish or become less effective as we age. An imbalance in the thyroid hormone can affect the body's ability to control its internal temperature and can cause hair loss or changes in hair quality, constipation, elevated cholesterol levels, depression, infertility, dry skin, weight gain and heart disease.

Sometimes the symptoms of thyroid imbalance may begin before blood levels change significantly enough to show up on lab tests. The balance of thyroid hormone is affected by nutrient deficiencies, stress and autoimmune dysfunction (where the body's own immune system attacks thyroid cells). Some studies suggest that older women with mild thyroid dysfunction and antibodies to the thyroid could be at a higher risk for complications of hypothyroidism, such as elevated cholesterol levels and heart disease.

Can We Quantify Aging?
Many of us quantify a person's age every day–either intentionally or unintentionally. We see someone and immediately make assumptions about his or her age and state

of health. We subconsciously review every aspect of the person: the quality of the skin; the degree of skin's sagging and the number of wrinkles; the color and quality of the hair, and the person's physique. We make judgments about their age.

But what do we really know about judging a person's physical appearance and how old they really are? Are there any specific lab tests that will tell us the real age of our bodies (often referred as our physiological age)? The short answer is no. However, evaluating the current state of our physical health can help determine how quickly we are aging. Measuring body fat percentage, blood pressure, inflammation and levels of blood sugar, insulin and hormones may help identify people at risk for developing many of the chronic illnesses associated with aging. Appraising the health of our bones, heart, blood vessels and brain may help make us aware of the damage that has already set in, enabling early intervention steps to slow down further damage. After all, the best course of action is always prevention!

Top 10 Ways to Slow Down the Aging Process

Everyone is looking for small steps to fight the signs of aging. Here are ten recommendations:

1. **Eat small meals every three hours**. This helps stabilize blood sugar levels throughout the day and reduce undue stress on your digestive system.

2. **Eat less sugar**. Sugar compromises the immune system, and high glycemic foods have been associated with cancer, diabetes and heart disease. Sugar can also bind and change the structure and function of proteins in the body causing extreme aging throughout the body. This process, called glycosylation, can damage enzymes, tissues and organs. Elevated blood sugar levels increase the risks of eye diseases, such as macular edema and diabetic retinopathy (which can lead to blindness); poor function or failure of the

kidneys, loss of limbs, and cardiovascular disease that leads to heart attack and stroke.

3. **Worry less about cholesterol**. Focusing solely on cholesterol tends to divert our attention away from the bigger picture when it comes to our heart disease risk. Elevated cholesterol does not occur in isolation. Healthy lifestyle, exercise and decreasing your body weight have a more profound effect on mortality than solely focusing on cholesterol levels.

4. **Quiet your mind**. Stress is a major component of many diseases. Cortisol, a stress hormone, ages the brain by literally shrinking the hippocampus, which is essential for memory and thinking. Cortisol causes you to gain weight around the middle and excess fat leads to inflammation. Excess cortisol can also cause an imbalance in blood sugar levels and predispose you to high blood pressure. Take a few minutes each day to quiet your mind with meditation, yoga, or deep breathing.

5. **Eat fish** or take a daily supplement (like fish oil) that contains omega-3 fatty acids. Fish oil supplements have been shown to lower blood pressure, improve one's mood, feed the brain, and reduce inflammation throughout the body.

6. **Stay connected**. Studies show that people who live the longest and lead the healthiest lives maintain connections to the community or a strong spiritual belief system. For more than two decades, research has shown that people with few social connections are more likely to have poor mental and physical health and die prematurely.

7. **Visit your physician for an annual wellness evaluation.** Knowing your current health status is the first step in creating your individual wellness plan.

8. **Exercise regularly**. You already knew that! Exercise is the single most important anti-aging tool you can apply. It strengthens bones, keeps muscles toned, increases circulation, reduces depression, lowers blood pressure, improves blood sugar levels, and increases oxygen to the brain. Why would you not use this one simple and effective anti-aging remedy? Get up and move!

9. **Lower inflammation**. When you injure a part of your body, chemicals in the body rush to the injured area, filling it with fluid and surrounding the injured areas with chemicals that fight infection as part of the healing process – this is a good thing! The problem is that many of us are battling chronic low-grade inflammation – this is <u>NOT</u> good! The negative aspect of this type of inflammation is that it can damage arteries and nerve cells, and is a leading contributor to every degenerative disease including Alzheimer's disease, diabetes, heart disease and obesity.

10. **Eat anti-inflammatory foods** like fish, berries, dark leafy greens, sweet potatoes and nuts. They contain phytonutrients and omega 3 fatty acids that reduce inflammation.

SHOULD WE SUPPLEMENT OUR DIET?

This is one of the major debates in the health, diet and nutrition field: to take or not to take. The studies seem to vary wildly, from supporting the use of supplements to indicating earlier deaths among those who do. Like everything else, I suspect that the answer lies in moderation and proper usage—taking vitamins and minerals only when indicated. Consider this scenario: what if physicians gave the same hypertensive medicine to all of their hypertensive patients? It would not work for every person and may even cause adverse reactions in some. Now imagine if this medication was given to all patients without evaluating their blood pressure–even more adverse reactions could be expected. The same is true for vitamin supplements – even though most of us consider them healthy and good for our bodies.

When vitamin studies are performed, the vitamin is often given to subjects without evaluating whether or not they specifically need that supplement. Even with naturally occurring nutrients, like the important mineral potassium, establishing individual requirements is imperative. Administering doses of potassium to an individual without establishing if he or she needs potassium replacement therapy could disrupt the heart beat; an improperly balanced potassium level could even prove fatal. In my opinion, vitamin therapy needs to be done by targeting the individual nutrient deficiencies or insufficiencies in the person being treated. While it has been established in the medical community that vitamin deficiencies can create disease states, it has never been established that vitamins can or should be used like pharmaceutical interventions.

In theory, it would be ideal to get all of our daily nutritional requirements from the foods we eat. It would be great if we all ate the recommended amounts of fruits, vegetables, protein and fats daily. It would be nice if our lives did not require more than the recommended daily allowance—that is, if we did not burn the candles at both ends and in the middle! It would be nice if most of our fast food choices didn't replace nutrients with saturated fats and sodium. Unfortunately, what would be ideal is not always the case for most people I have met in my personal life or treated as patients.

Even if it were true that eating a balanced diet would give us all of the vitamins and minerals we needed without supplements, research shows that most people do not eat a good, balanced diet. Furthermore, stress, illnesses, alcohol, smoking and even physical exertion use up the vitamins in our bodies, and may even deplete some of them so that we need to take a multi-vitamin.

So my response as to whether or not you should take a multi-vitamin is this: If you eat a perfectly balanced meal every day, stay young and have no stress in your life, then a multivitamin may not be for you. However, if your body decides to age faster than you would like; you have days when a vegetable is a foreign object, and you find yourself constantly resisting the urge to scream at the top of your lungs because something is going contrary to the way you expected, then taking a good multivitamin may be worth considering.

So what is a good multivitamin? Are they all made the same? How many should you take? What is the RDA (recommended daily allowance) of nutrients? Can you take too many vitamins? What does a good multivitamin do? In the next section, many of these common questions about multivitamins are answered.

RDA

The United States recommended daily allowance (RDA) is the daily amount of a protein, vitamin, or mineral that the Food and Drug Administration (FDA) has established as sufficient to maintain the nutritional health of persons in various age groups and categories. RDA is the minimum amount of a given nutrient needed to ward off serious deficiencies and disease, not the minimum needed to maintain optimal health. It is helpful to keep in mind that the goal of any regulatory agency is to establish what is needed to keep the general population disease-free. The goal of optimal health is not their primary concern, and because individual needs differ, it is best to treat each person as an individual and examine their specific needs.

Studies show that even mild nutrient deficiencies can compromise function, even if they have not yet overtly caused a major disease.

Yet, the simple rule of supply and demand seems to apply to the body. If demands go up, supply must go up, or deficiencies will follow. For example, recent studies suggest that our requirement for vitamin D may be significantly higher than the currently established RDA.

In Table 5, you'll see a list of the suggested U.S. RDAs for most nutrients based on a 2,000-calorie a day diet for adults and children over the age of four. The chart shows the minimum recommended amount of specific nutrients needed so that a body can avoid diseases.

Table 5: Recommended U.S. RDA Amounts:

Nutrient	Unit of Measure	RDA Daily Values
Vitamin A	International Unit (IU)	5,000
Vitamin C	milligrams (mg)	60
Calcium	milligrams (mg)	1,000
Iron	milligrams (mg)	18
Vitamin D	International Unit (IU)	400
Vitamin E	International Unit (IU)	30
Vitamin K	Micrograms (μg)	80
Thiamin	milligrams (mg)	1.5
Riboflavin	milligrams (mg)	1.7
Niacin	milligrams (mg)	20
Vitamin B_6	milligrams (mg)	2.0
Folate	Micrograms (μg)	400
Vitamin B_{12}	Micrograms (μg)	6.0
Biotin	Micrograms (μg)	300
Pantothenic acid	milligrams (mg)	10
Phosphorus	milligrams (mg)	1,000
Iodine	Micrograms (μg)	150
Magnesium	milligrams (mg)	400
Zinc	milligrams (mg)	15

Selenium	Micrograms (µg)	70
Copper	milligrams (mg)	2.0
Manganese	milligrams (mg)	2.0
Chromium	Micrograms (µg)	120
Molybdenum	Micrograms (µg)	75
Chloride	milligrams (mg)	3,400

Believe it or not, many of us consistently fall short of the minimum recommended daily requirements. Lifestyle choices may place an even greater demand on our bodies, leaving us vulnerable to sickness and disease if we don't replenish the nutrients.

So how do we decide whether we need to take a multivitamin? First, know that no vitamin, herb or medicine takes the place of making healthier lifestyle choices. Taking a multivitamin is not a license to practice poor lifestyle habits with the expectation that you are instantly protected against potentially adverse outcomes of our choices. *Vitamins are designed to complement a healthy lifestyle– not create one.* Thus, it is important to take stock of your life, pantry and medicine cabinet.

First, take an honest look at your life. Does your life run 100 miles an hour in the fast lane? You may have noticed the warning signs. You feel that there are not enough hours in the day to get things done. You know everyone is conspiring to drive you crazy. You are short tempered, moody or just plain anxious most of the time. You can't remember the last time you took a vacation, or even time for a deep breath. Stress is the one of the greatest drain on our body's energy and resources.

Take stock of your pantry. Does it look like the chips and cookie aisle in the grocery store? Does your refrigerator include more leftover fast food take-out containers or fresh vegetables and fruits?

How much do you know about the contents of your medicine cabinet? Does it contain medications that could interfere with absorption of nutrients and contribute to vitamin deficiencies? Are you on medications that could have possible interactions or side effects with your vitamins? For example, if you are on a blood thinner, you may want to avoid supplements with vitamin K, which can potentially interfere with the effects of this medication.

If you discover that you are running on all cylinders, yet you are not feeling as well as you would like and there are no contraindications, then you may want to supplement your diet with a quality multivitamin that meets or exceeds the RDA. However, using mega doses of vitamins without a sufficient indication of a deficiency may not be beneficial and could be potentially harmful. Remember the body tends to strive for balance, and large doses of one vitamin may cause an imbalance in another and create unwanted effects.

The Profile of the Multivitamin
Here is a quick breakdown of some of the basic ingredients in the average multivitamin and the effects on the body. While the overt signs of deficiencies are well known, the subtle signs of insufficiency (intake that is not sufficient for a person's lifestyle) are harder to notice. This information is not an all-inclusive look at vitamins but rather just the beginning. It's best to pay attention to your own body and recognize when it is off-balance.

Vitamin A (also known as retinol): This fat-soluble vitamin produces the light-sensitive tissue lining the inner surface of the eyeball that enables good vision, especially in low-light situations. Vitamin A comes in two major forms in food: retinol, absorbed primarily from animal products, and carotenes, obtained primarily from colorful fruits and vegetables. Carotene is converted to vitamin A in the body.

Symptoms of Vitamin A deficiency can range from dry eyes, difficulty seeing in dim light or night, or complete blindness. Individuals with this deficiency are also prone to infections that may be fatal, and it can also lead to slow bone development in children. People who avoid animal products, such as liver and dairy products and do not consume a variety of colored vegetables, such as kale and carrots are susceptible to vitamin A deficiencies. Individuals with mal-absorption issues can also be at increased risk for vitamin A deficiency. Individuals with hypothyroidism (low functioning thyroid) may have a problem efficiently converting carotene in the body to vitamin A and could be at risk.

Because vitamin A is fat soluble (stores itself in fat), it can accumulate in the body and possibly cause toxicity if high quantities are ingested. Signs and symptoms of toxicity are abdominal pain, headaches, irritability, anemia and hair loss. Excessive vitamin A can also contribute to an increased risk of fractures possibly due to interference with vitamin D, an important component of bone health. Here is an example where balance, rather than random supplementation, is imperative.

Table 6: Recommended Dietary Allowance (RDA) for Vitamin A, according to the Institute of Health

Age (yrs)	Children	Men	Women	Pregnancy	Lactation
1 to 3	1,000				
4 to 8	1,333				
9 to 13	2,000				
14 to 18		3,000	2,330	2,500	4,000
19+		3,000	2,330	2,565	4,335

Vitamin B1, Thiamine, like the other B-complex vitamins, is water-soluble, so the body can excrete it, rather than storing it in fat tissue. It is an essential vitamin, meaning it is not made by the body, but must be obtained from foods. It is found in

beans, cereal grains, meats and nuts. It is required for the synthesis of ATP, the energy that fuels every cell in the body. Deficiencies are rare in developed countries because most foods are enriched with vitamin B1. However, in cases where absorption and storage of nutrients is limited, such as Crohn's disease, alcohol abuse and conditions requiring the use of prescription diuretics or dialysis, deficiencies are more common and can cause beriberi, a disease of the peripheral nervous system that primarily affects the function of the heart and causes paralysis or pain in the extremities. Vitamin B1 has been used therapeutically to treat diabetic kidney impairment, dementia and immune system insufficiencies.

Vitamin B3 comes in several different forms: nictonic acid (niacin), niacinamide and inositol hexanicotinate. Niacin can be found in foods including brewer's yeast, beets, liver, peanuts, sunflower seeds, and fish such as salmon and tuna. It plays an important role in helping the body to make sex and stress hormones, and like other B vitamins it helps the body convert carbohydrates to energy. People with conditions that cause mal-absorption and those who consume excess amounts of alcohol can become deficient in niacin. Signs and symptoms of deficiency include fatigue, depression, indigestion, canker sores, and a swollen, bright red tongue. Severe niacin deficiency can lead to a disease called pellagra that is characterized by skin changes, severe nerve and mental dysfunction, and diarrhea.

Niacin has been used to treat high cholesterol as both pharmaceutical and nutritional therapy for many years. However, it is imperative to follow a physician's advice when using high, therapeutic levels of niacin. High levels have the potential to cause liver damage and possibly elevate blood sugar levels in people with Type 2 diabetes. Some preliminary research suggests that niacin may be helpful in improving

arthritic symptoms, reducing the risk of heart attack or strokes, delaying the onset of Type 1 diabetes, and lowering the chances of developing cataracts.

One of the most common side effects of taking supplemental niacin is a bright red flushing and tingling sensation in face and chest. Individuals with stomach ulcers or liver or kidney disease should not take niacin supplements. Niacin can potentially interact with blood pressure or cholesterol medications. Niacin may also affect the levels of certain seizure and blood thinner medications.

Vitamin B12 is generally found in animal products such as fish, meat, eggs and milk, and is water-soluble. People who do not consume animal products, like strict vegetarians and vegans, may need to take a B12 supplement to avoid the risk of deficiency. Older individuals with atrophic gastritis are also at risk because their bodies produce lower amounts of stomach acid and have difficulty absorbing vitamin B12 from foods. Other conditions that may contribute to vitamin B12 deficiency are Crohn's disease, pernicious anemia and celiac disease— which all affect absorption. Certain medications such as H2 blockers (used to decrease acid production in the stomach), some antibiotics and Metformin, (commonly prescribed for Type 2 diabetes), can also decrease the absorption of B12.

Vitamin B12 is a prerequisite for the production of healthy myelin, the fatty sheath that insulates nerve fibers, as well as the synthesis of the red blood cells. Deficiencies may result in anemia and nerve damage leading to neuropathies. A lack of B12 can also contribute to increased homocysteine levels, which may increase risks of cardiovascular disease.

If the deficiency is treated, the accompanying anemia and neuropathy can be corrected while boosting moods and energy levels. Vitamin B12 supplementation has not been shown to cause any serious adverse effects in healthy individuals.

Biotin, or B5, is needed by most organisms to survive, but can only be made by bacteria, yeast and certain plants. In the human body, the "good bacteria" are responsible for the synthesis of biotin. It can also be found in small quantities in certain foods like brewer's yeast, liver, egg yolks and green leafy vegetables. Anti-seizure medications can lead to depletion of biotin. Taking large dosages of vitamin B5 can compete with the absorption of biotin and contribute to a deficiency as well.

Biotin plays an important role in the metabolism of fatty acids and the formation of glucose. Recent studies point towards biotin's role in speeding up the replication our DNA. Biotin can help support the formation of new cells especially those that divide rapidly, like the skin. One study revealed biotin levels were significantly lower in individuals with Type 2 diabetes than other healthy patients. After one month of biotin supplementation, the patients' fasting blood sugar levels improved by 45 percent.

Signs of deficiency include hair loss and a red scaly rash around mouth, eyes, nose and genital area. A few studies suggest that biotin may also be helpful to strengthen brittle nails. Biotin is not known to be toxic and seems to be well tolerated even in large amounts.

Vitamin D is fat-soluble and found naturally in foods like fatty fish including salmon, tuna and mackerel, as well as liver and egg yolks. The primary source of vitamin D comes from fortified foods and sunlight absorbed through the skin and converted in the body.

Individuals at risk for vitamin D deficiency reside in Northern climates, have darker complexions due to a lack of absorption of sunshine, and older individuals who have a decreased ability to convert vitamin D from the sun. Obese people are also at risk because the fat-soluble vitamin has more opportunities to bind with fat cells, preventing it from entering the bloodstream. Medications that can interfere with the absorption and function of vitamin D include steroids, medications for weight loss that prevent fat absorption, and certain anti-seizure medications. The best way to evaluate for vitamin D deficiency is to measure the levels of D25 in the blood. Blood levels less than 32ng/ml are considered Vitamin D deficient.

A deficiency in Vitamin D can make us more vulnerable to viral and other infectious diseases. Recent studies suggest it regulates the immune system, possibly decreasing the risk for autoimmune diseases and certain cancers. Recent studies also support the role of Vitamin D to help maintain a healthy blood pressure and suggest it may be an important part to low a person's risk of developing Type 2 diabetes. Vitamin D also is crucial to maintaining healthy bones. Vitamin D deficiency can also be responsible for significant musculoskeletal pain (sore muscles and achy bones). Individuals with the diagnosis of fibromyalgia should have their vitamin D level checked to see if a deficiency may be contributing to their symptomology.

As with all fat-soluble vitamins, it is possible to have too much vitamin D in the bloodstream because it may accumulate in fat cells. Signs of toxicity are nausea, vomiting, weakness, disorientation and constipation. Excessive amounts of vitamin D can also damage kidneys and disturb heart rhythms. Again, recall the importance of an evaluation before taking high dosages of any nutrient. The dose of 400 IU of vitamin D, found in most multivitamins, is not usually enough to cause toxicity in healthy individuals.

Vitamin E is fat-soluble and represents a family of antioxidants including tocopherols and tocotrienols that help to prevent damage caused by free radicals. Vitamin E is most active in the lipid or fatty portions of the cells and helps maintain the integrity of the cell membranes. The tocopherols are the form most likely to be labeled as vitamin E in a multivitamin. There are four forms of tocopherols: alpha, beta, gamma and delta. Alpha tocopherol is the form found in the highest concentration in the body, while gamma tocopherol is the form found in high concentration in foods. When it is listed on supplement labels, the natural form of vitamin E obtained from foods is called d-alpha tocopherol. The synthetic laboratory equivalent is listed as dl-alpha tocopherol. The synthetic form of this vitamin has approximately half of the potency of its natural form.

Adequate intake and absorption of vitamin E can reduce the risks of many conditions, including cardiovascular disease, impaired immunity, cancer and cataracts. Vitamin E retards the oxidation of the LDL (bad) cholesterol, reducing the chances that it will cause plaque build-up within the arterial walls. The Cambridge Heart Antioxidant Study (CHAOS) followed more than 2,000 heart disease patients who took 400 to 800 IU of vitamin E daily. The study found that the patients had 75 percent fewer heart attacks than those taking a placebo. Vitamin E may also protect the brain by preventing memory loss and dementia. Studies have shown Vitamin E decreases the ability of the platelets to bind. Individuals on certain medications such as blood thinners should consult with their physician before taking this multivitamin.

Vitamin E can be found in wheat germ, nuts (peanuts and almonds), seeds and their oils (e.g., sunflower or safflower) and, of course, fortified foods. The diet of most Americans provides less than the recommended daily allowance so supplements may be needed.

Vitamin K is required for the production of prothrombin, a necessary component for blood clotting. Main food sources of vitamin K come from green leafy vegetables such as kale, Swiss chard, parsley, and broccoli. Bacteria living in the gut also produce vitamin K. There is a concern among physicians that prolonged use of certain antibiotics can create a deficiency by eliminating the bacteria responsible for the formation of vitamin K and lead to abnormal bleeding and/or internal bleeding.

In addition to the important role vitamin K serves in proper blood clotting, studies support an additional role in bone formation that possibly decreases the risk of osteoporosis. The cells in the bone responsible for bone formation are called osteoblasts. These cells produce a protein called osteocalcin that is an important part of this process. To be fully functional or work properly osteocalcin needs to have additional groups (called carboxyl groups) added to its main structure. Vitamin K helps with this process and many studies show that osteocalcin without the carboxyl group is not as effective in bone formation.

Osteocalcin also acts as a hormone for the pancreas to help regulate insulin and blood sugar levels. In fact studies show that individuals with higher osteocalcin levels have regular levels of glucose (sugar), insulin, and a lower risk for insulin resistance. As you can see, the body with its series of checks and balances works in perfect synchrony.

Inappropriate calcium deposits in the walls of the blood vessels can lead to the narrowing and hardening of these walls and increases the risk of strokes, heart attacks and peripheral vascular disease. Some studies suggest that vitamin K may help prevent this deposition of calcium.

If you are taking blood-thinning drugs such as Coumadin or Warfarin, you need to talk to your doctor about consuming vitamin K through food and supplements. Some studies suggest that long term use of Warfarin could increase risk of osteoporosis so be sure to discuss and follow up with your physician regarding your bone health.

Calcium and Magnesium are two of the important minerals used by the body. Approximately 99 percent of the body's calcium is found in bone and teeth, with only one percent found in blood and tissue. It is so important for calcium levels to be maintained within a certain range; if daily intake is not adequate, the body will take calcium from these available resources.

Calcium plays an important role in the contraction and relaxation of blood vessels and muscles. It also helps activate the breakdown of sugar storage in the muscles to provide them with energy and activate blood clotting.

Calcium may be the most common mineral, but many diets still lack the minimum amount. You need different levels of calcium at different stages of your life, especially young children and women. Below is a chart that offers the recommended daily allowances for each life stage for children, men and women.

Table 7: Recommended Dietary Allowance (RDA) for Calcium

Life Stage	Age	Males (mg/day)	Females (mg/day)
Infants	0-6 months	200 (AI)	200 (AI)
Infants	6-12 months	260 (AI)	260 (AI)
Children	1-3 years	700	700
Children	4-8 years	1,000	1,000
Children	9-13 years	1,300	1,300
Adolescents	14-18 years	1,300	1,300
Adults	19-50 years	1,000	1,000
Adults	51-70 years	1,000	1,200
Adults	71 years and older	1,200	1,200
Pregnancy	14-18 years	-	1,300
Pregnancy	19-50 years	-	1,000
Breastfeeding	14-18 years	-	1,300
Breastfeeding	19-50 years	-	1,000

Different conditions can affect calcium levels in the body. They include low vitamin D or magnesium levels, kidney failure, and abnormal parathyroid glands (glands located in the thyroid gland that help control calcium levels in body). It is also interesting to note that some studies suggest that a high sodium intake can lead to an increased calcium loss in the urine, which may increase the rate of bone loss. Remember one of the primary reservoirs for calcium in the body are bones.

Believe it or not, several studies suggest individuals with a higher dietary calcium intake have lower risks of kidney stones than those with a lower intake. Researchers suggest that increased calcium excretion caused by high sodium in the diet may play a larger role in the formation of kidney stones than calcium intake itself.

The major source of dietary calcium in the U.S. comes from dairy products and fortified foods. Vegetables, such as kale, spinach, beans and tofu, provide vegan sources of calcium. One concern about consuming calcium from some of these vegetables is that they naturally contain phytochemicals that may prevent the complete absorption of calcium. Still, most health and nutrition professionals would agree that the majority of a person's calcium should come from diet.

Because calcium is bulky, it is not possible for a multivitamin to contain the complete recommended daily allowance; therefore, many people supplement their diet with additional calcium. Calcium carbonate is the most common and economical form of supplemental calcium, but is not the most absorbable and must be taken with food to increase absorbability. Also, calcium supplements can potentially interfere with the absorption of some medications so it is recommended that it be taken about two hours apart from other medications such as thyroid and certain blood pressure medications.

Also, caution should be exercised when taking calcium as a supplement; it is possible to develop hypercalcemia (too much calcium in the blood). Symptoms include nausea, abdominal pain, vomiting, constipation, increased urination and dry mouth. Severe toxicity can result in confusion, weakness and even coma and must be treated promptly. Fortunately, this condition is rare unless some disease process is involved. It is more common to find that many individuals do not get the RDA of calcium through the diet.

Iron is the most common deficiency in the diet, not only in the U.S., but worldwide. It can result in anemia, or decreased red blood cell production, as well as an increase in lactic acid formation, which affects the body's ability to maintain a normal temperature when exposed to cold. Inadequate intake of iron can result in complications during pregnancy. Iron also plays a role in the formation of certain neurotransmitters in the brain, and deficiencies can lead to fatigue and poor cognitive function. Some studies suggest that iron deficiency in the central nervous system may play a role in a condition called Restless Leg Syndrome.

Groups vulnerable for iron deficiencies include infants and children up to 4 years of age, adolescents, women who are menstruating and pregnant, gastric bypass patients and vegetarians (who often get their iron from plant-based foods and is not well absorbed compared to iron from meat sources). Other conditions associated with low-iron levels are acute or chronic blood loss and celiac disease.

As with calcium, you need different amounts of iron at different stages of your life. Below is a breakdown of iron levels required at varying ages.

Table 8: Recommended Dietary Allowances (RDA) for Iron

Life Stage	Age	Males (mg/day)	Females (mg/day)
Infants	0-6 months	0.27 (AI)	0.27 (AI)
Infants	7-12 months	11	11
Children	1-3 years	7	7
Children	4-8 years	10	10
Children	9-13 years	8	8
Adolescents	14-18 years	11	15
Adults	19-50 years	8	18
Adults	51 years and older	8	8
Pregnancy	All ages	-	27
Breastfeeding	18 years and younger	-	10
Breastfeeding	19 years and older	-	9

Accidental iron overdose is the leading cause of poisoning fatalities in children under the age of 6. Be sure to consult with your child's pediatrician regarding dosage before administering iron and always keep out of the reach of children. Iron overdose is a medical emergency, and it can lead to organ injury or failure, or even death. Even at dosages for the therapeutic treatment of deficiency, taking iron can cause symptoms of nausea, abdominal discomfort and constipation.

Due to the potential for inflammation and toxicity caused by excessive iron amounts, it is important to have your iron levels checked before taking any supplementation. Many multivitamins have iron-free choice to accommodate individuals who should avoid additional iron supplementation, such as healthy men and people with a genetic condition called hemochromatosis (excess iron is present in the body). Also, the cause of the deficiency may need further exploration by your physician.

Some Helpful Hints in Selecting Multivitamins:

1. If you have a challenge swallowing tablets, then try the soft gel vitamins. Avoid taking vitamins with coffee because it can hinder the absorption of some vitamins and minerals.

2. Be sure the vitamins address your specific needs and age. For example, do you need a vitamin with or without iron? Are you nursing or pregnant and require additional nutrients?

3. If a vitamin causes an upset stomach, look at the mineral components, such as the calcium and magnesium. Are they oxides or carbonates? Many individuals find they can tolerate minerals chelated to citrate or gluconate. For example, if

you are taking a vitamin with calcium carbonate and magnesium oxide, try one with calcium citrate and magnesium citrate.

4. Finally, if you have any concerns consult your physician.

A multivitamin may boost deficiency levels in your diet, but can other supplements give you the upper hand in the fight against aging? Here is a look at some other anti-aging supplements:

1. **Resveratrol** is a powerful antioxidant that can be found in such foods as grapes (skin only), grape juice (purple), blueberries, bilberries, cranberries and wine. The amount of resveratrol found in these foods varies widely depending on geographical region where they were grown and the fermentation time of wine.

   Resveratrol came to the attention of the scientific community when laboratory studies showed that it prevented the growth of human cancer cells in the breast, colon, prostate, pancreas and thyroid. Animal studies reinforced the findings of inhibitory effects of cancer cells in the breast, colon and esophagus (Cancer Res. 2001;61(20):7456-7463., Carcinogenesis. 2002;23(9):1531-1536, Carcinogenesis. 2000;21(8):1619-1622).

   Additional lab studies showed that resveratrol prevented platelets from sticking together; enhanced the production of nitric oxide, causing the relaxation of blood vessels and decreased the production of inflammatory substances, thereby having potential cardio-protective effects. (Anticancer Res. 2004;24(5A):2783-2840, Blood Cells Mol Dis. 2000;26(2):144-150, Clin Chim Acta. 1995;235(2):207-219. Biochem Biophys Res Commun.

2003;311(2):546-552., J Biol Chem. 2004;279(21):22727-22737. J Agric Food Chem. 1999;47(12):4842-4846.). If we are able to decrease the formation of clots by making platelets less sticky, maintain healthy blood pressure by keeping blood vessels relaxed, and decrease plaque formation by decreasing inflammatory response, then we can certainly see how this could go a long way to keeping us heart healthy.

Recently, it has been shown that caloric restriction has the ability to prolong lifespan in many species including mammals. The mechanism of action seems to be activation of a particular enzyme known as the Sir2. In lab tests on lower life forms, resveratrol was shown to extend life through a mechanism similar to caloric restriction. It seems to activate enzymes homologous to the Sir 2 enzyme. In test tube studies, resveratrol increased the activity of a similar human enzyme called Sirtuin 1, or SIRT1. It is unclear if this would have the same effect in vivo (a living person).

The concern with resveratrol is that the same levels required to achieve the results in the lab were not achievable in human serum after oral doses were administered. However, a recent study in mice using smaller doses delivered orally showed changes in genes expression similar to effects of caloric restriction (Barger JL, Kayo T, Vann JM, et al.) A low dose of dietary resveratrol partially mimics caloric restriction and retards aging parameters in mice (PLoS One. 2008;3(6):e2264.). Currently, resveratrol is not known to have adverse effects on humans, although safety in pregnancy and lactation has not been established.

2. **Coenzyme CoQ10:** Coenzyme Q10 (CoQ10) is a fat-soluble substance made by the body, but also found in foods. It is found in virtually all cell membranes throughout the body including the inner mitochondrial membrane. One function of the mitochondria is to help convert food into energy the body can use. CoQ10 also functions as a powerful fat-soluble anti-oxidant.

    As people age or experience extreme stress, CoQ10 levels can drop. Low levels are also found in diseases such as diabetes, congestive heart failure and cancer. Cholesterol lowering medications can also decrease levels of CoQ10. This drop can contribute to the loss of efficiency and capacity of the cells to protect the body. This is why supplements and especially the reduced form of CoQ10 called Ubiquinol are one of the more efficient anti-aging agents that replace lost CoQ10 in the cells.

3. **Essential Fatty Acids, like Omega-3s, from flax seed and fish oil**s: Omega-3 is an essential fatty acid that is vital to ensure proper heath and promote anti-aging. These essential fatty acids promote healthy cells, and proper development and the smooth functioning of the brain and the nervous system. Essential fatty acids help regulate blood pressure, blood viscosity, inflammatory and immune system responses and cholesterol levels in the body. However, many people lack this very important nutrient in their daily diet. It is recommended that supplements for anti-aging and overall health should be taken together along with a proper diet. Look for an Omega-3 supplement that contains all three essential oils – flax oil, fish oil and borage oil – in one formula with a recommended amount of 1,000 mg per day.

**

UPDATE:

During her evaluation, Kate's levels of hs-CRP, cholesterol, and cortisol were slightly elevated. All of these values could be attributed to her former eating habits and lifestyle. As we have learned, diet, stress and a lack of exercise can adversely affect each of these factors. The changes that Kate instituted throughout her treatment will go a long way to improve these values and decrease her risk of chronic illnesses.

Kate's thyroid function was borderline normal. Her stress level contributed to elevated cortisol levels, which may have been interfering with the function of the thyroid hormone. It was important to continually monitor the thyroid function as Kate instituted lifestyle changes to reduce stress and improve her responses. Her blood test did not reveal an autoimmune issue with her thyroid. Kate's sex hormone levels were also normal.

Simple STEP 8
Anti-Aging Skin Care

Our skin is our largest vital organ and first line of defense. It helps protect us from the environment, maintain our body temperature, and serves as the primary source of synthesis of vitamin D. Our skin is made up of two primary layers: the epidermis and dermis. The epidermis is the top layer of the skin. Epidermis is waterproof and helps retain moisture in the skin. This layer of skin also contains cells that are part of the skin's immune system. Other cells in this layer called melanocytes produce the melanin responsible for pigmentation of skin and filtering harmful ultraviolet radiation from sunlight.

The dermis is the second layer of skin and is made up of a thick layer of fibrous and elastic tissue that is approximately 80 percent collagen. It helps the skin to maintain its elasticity, strength and smoothness. Elastin is another protein present in the dermis and helps to provide elasticity to the skin through its interaction with collagen. The dermis also contains nerve endings, some hair follicles, oil secreting glands (sebaceous) and blood vessels. The dermis also supplies nourishment to the epidermis. There is a layer under the skin known as the subcutaneous layer. This layer contains adipose tissue (fat), sweat glands and blood vessels. It forms a cushion underneath the skin that prevents it from falling onto the bone. All three layers work together to give our skin a smooth, youthful appearance.

Also present in the skin are substances known as GAGS (Glycosaminoglycans) and proteoglycans. These are specialized sugars with the ability to hold many times their actual weight in water. GAGS help the skin seal in moisture and appear plump and well nourished.

Visible aging of the skin can start as early as age 25. These changes begin to accelerate in our 40s when hormonal changes and decreasing hormonal levels begin to play a significant role. The skin can be affected by many factors including aging, environmental changes, poor nutrition, medications, stress and hereditary factors. As we get older, the skin cells divide slower and the top layer of skin gets 10 percent thinner every 10 years. The number of melanin cells in the top layer shrinks. This causes the skin to appear thinner and more translucent. Another noticeable change is the formation of excessive pigmented areas known as age or liver spots in the epidermis layer. This is usually secondary to damage from excessive sun exposure.

Changes are also taking place in the dermis. The blood vessels in the dermis become more fragile and rupture easily causing skin bruises. This along with thinning of the skin could worsen the appearance of those dreaded under eye circles that make us look tired and older than we really are. The oil producing glands become less active. The amount of moisture holding GAGS in the skin decreases leaving the skin drier, looser and less plump.

Environmental conditions like excessive sun exposure, poor nutrition and smoking can speed up the loss of collagen and elastin and accelerate the aging process (*Photochem Photobiol*, 1993 Dec;58(6):841-4.). UVA rays in sunlight weaken collagen and cause the excessive production of abnormal elastin. The exposure to free radicals, generated by smoking and excessive sun exposure, causes a decrease in collagen production while activating the production of an enzyme known as metalloproteinase. This enzyme breaks down damaged collagen in preparation for removal and remodeling. However, since collagen production has been decreased, much of the collagen produced is abnormal and does not possess the strength and elasticity of the original level. The fatty subcutaneous layer thins out and makes the skin looser. Combined with gravity's effects and habitual facial expressions, our skin can be left with distinct wrinkle patterns (crow's feet or laugh lines), loose sagging skin, loss of facial volume, a dry, uneven skin tone, hyperpigmentation and broken capillaries.

Now that we have a very basic understanding of what happens to the skin as we age, we are now in a position to understand the many options science and research have provided us to slow down and improve the visible signs of aging. We are bombarded on a daily basis with lotions and portions that claim to not only stop the aging process, but also magically return our skin to the look of our youth. What is fact and what is fiction? Is it even possible to affect change with topical creams? What other technology is available to help us reduce the visible signs of aging?

The first step in developing a daily skin care regimen is to determine your skin type and condition. This is an opportunity to determine if there is any evidence of sun damage. Do you notice wrinkles when your muscles are relaxed or are they only noticeable during expressions? Is there evidence of photo damage such as hyperpigmentation spots?

1. **Determine Your Skin Type**: The key to developing a good skin care regimen that works for you is to determine your individual skin type. You can try a home evaluation test first. If you have any doubts or questions, visit to your dermatologist or skin care professional for additional testing.

To analyze your skin at home, try the these steps:

> Wash your face with a mild lathering facial cleanser.
> Wait for at least half an hour to allow the oil time to return to the skin.
> Examine your skin in a mirror under good daylight or a white-light.

Check your skin condition against one of the following skin types below:

NORMAL SKIN:

Normal skin is balanced. It is not too oily or too dry. It appears soft, smooth and even toned with small to medium poor size. Normal skin usually consists of the following characteristics:

> You will feel smooth and comfortable after cleansing. You can either use facial wash with water or cleansing bar with water or cream cleanser.
> Your skin still appears fresh and clean by midday.
> You will only experience occasional outbreaks of acne and pimples, perhaps before or during your menstrual period, or when you are under a lot of stress.
> You will have no problems using a facial toner.
> Your skin feels very comfortable after applying rich night cream.

DRY SKIN:

This skin type is under active and may feel tight and look flaky. It is sensitive to cold weather and loses moisture easily. It can be easily irritated. Dry skin can look older and have a tendency to develop fine lines around the eyes. Dry skin rarely suffers acne outbreaks.

Dry skin would usually have most of the following characteristics:

After cleansing with facial wash or cleansing bar and water, your skin feels tight, as though it is too small for your face.

> ➢ Your skin feels relatively comfortable after cleansing with cream cleanser.
> ➢ Flaky patches starts to appear by midday.
> ➢ You have few experiences with outbreaks of acne and pimples.
> ➢ Your skin will sting after applying facial toner.
> ➢ Your skin will feel very comfortable after applying rich night cream.

Conditions that can exacerbate dry skin types include:
- Incorrect use of cosmetics
- Not thoroughly washing your skin
- The condition of your thyroid gland
- Skin Aging
- Genetic predisposition
- Certain medications or over the counter products such as antihistamines

OILY SKIN:
Oily skin is under active and may have a shiny complexion. It has a tendency towards larger pores and is acne prone. Oily skin has most of the following characteristics:

> ➢ Your skin feels fine and quite comfortable after cleansing with facial wash or cleansing bar and water.
> ➢ Your skin feels quite oily after cleansing with cream cleanser.
> ➢ Your skin will most likely appear shiny by midday.
> ➢ You may experience frequent outbreaks of acne and pimples.
> ➢ Your skin feels fresh after applying facial toner.

➢ Your skin feels very oily after applying rich night cream.

There are certain factors that can exacerbate oily skin types. These include:

- Aggressive cleaning with cosmetics that contain irritating ingredients
- Overactive sebaceous glands
- Stress
- Hormonal disorders
- Genetic predisposition

Uncovering the reason for overabundant oil production is an important step towards improving oily skin. See your dermatologist for further evaluation.

COMBINATION SKIN:

A combination skin has oiliness in the T-zone (across your forehead and down your nose and chin area) and dryness on the cheeks. There are occasional acne outbreaks in the oily areas. A combination skin would usually have most of the following characteristics:

➢ Your skin feels dry in some areas and smooth in others after cleansing with facial wash or cleansing bar and water.
➢ Your skin feels oily in some areas and smooth in others after cleansing with cream cleanser.
➢ Your skin may appear shiny in some areas, especially the T-zone, by midday.
➢ You may experience frequent outbreaks of acne and pimples, especially in the T-zone.
➢ Your skin will feel fresh in some areas, but stings in

other areas after applying facial toner.

- ➤ Your skin will feel very oily in the T-zone and comfortable on the cheeks after applying rich night cream.

Uncovering the reason for overabundant oil production and the cause of dryness is an important step towards improving combination skin. Aggressive washing with skin care products containing irritating ingredients can stimulate excessive oil production in the central portion of the face and dry out the skin on other portions.

SENSITIVE SKIN:

Sensitive skin is delicate and may over react to external factors such as soaps, creams and other topical products. There may be a tendency towards redness and broken capillaries. Sensitive skin would usually have most of the following characteristics:

- ➤ Your skin feels dry and itchy in some places after cleansing with facial wash or cleansing bar and water.
- ➤ Your skin feels sometimes uncomfortable or itchy after cleansing with cream cleanser.
- ➤ Flaky patches and some redness may appear by midday.
- ➤ You may experience occasional outbreaks of acne and pimples.
- ➤ Your skin will sting and itch after applying facial toner.

Once you have determined your skin type, you are now ready to choose the right skin care product for your skin. A dermatologist may use special tools to help determine the moisture content in your skin and evaluate any signs of sun damage. Prescription strength or medical grade skin products may be prescribed. Your physician may also go over with you other interventions that may help you to achieve the look you want, and also help you to put a plan in place to reduce future damage.

How important is anti-aging skin care?

Protecting your skin from the elements starts as early as childhood. Wearing sunscreen and hats while in the sun for an extended length of time is probably the single most important anti-aging step to limit sun damage. The second most important thing, in my opinion, is to stay well hydrated.

The re-hydration of the skin starts from within the body. Anti-aging skin care is most effective when an outer form of moisture is combined with inner moisture that is natural and self-replenishing. A simply regime of 6 to 8 glasses of water each day goes a long way to hydrating the body and the skin. Hydrated skin appears smoother and younger.

Fortunately, for those of us who didn't follow the sunscreen regime in our childhood and suffered a few sunburns, some anti-aging topical ingredients show great promise to enhance the appearance and texture of our skin. Some may even help reverse the visible signs of damage already inflicted. Products and procedures that encourage higher cellular turnover rate and enhance collagen production can assist the skin to hold onto moisture and improve its appearance, tone and texture. Skin appears more even toned, smoother and less pigmented.

When choosing the right serum or cream, it's important to look for specific active ingredients in the product. Don't get distracted with expensive creams and packaging. Read the product's ingredients and find the vital nutrients that will help nourish and restore your skin. Here's what to look for:

VITAMIN C

Vitamin C is necessary for the formation of collagen in the tissues. Humans lack the ability to produce vitamin C naturally in the body and must obtained it through foods. Research has shown that oral vitamin C supplementation does not increase the concentration of this important vitamin. However, studies show that topical application of vitamin C is one of the most effective ways to boost collagen formation in the skin.

Vitamin C is also a potent anti-oxidant that helps to neutralize free radicals in the skin. Free radicals are unstable, reactive molecules that form during the body's normal metabolic reactions. They need to bind to another molecule to stabilize. When free radicals bind to collagen, they form breaks in the collagen molecule that change the chemical structure and cause it to become more disorganized. This new form of collagen loses its tensile strength and makes the skin look saggy and wrinkly.

Several studies have shown that vitamin C can reduce the appearance of fine lines and wrinkles in as little as 12 weeks. Skin tone and clarity, acne and even age spots have also shown significant improvement. Topical Vitamin C provides multiple benefits to the skin including:

- Moisturizes
- Encourages growth of collagen
- Softens
- Exfoliates and cleanses
- Helps remove wrinkles
- Improves skin tone and clarity

NIACINAMIDE

A derivative of Vitamin B3 (niacin) has shown in several studies to offer anti-aging benefits when applied topically to the skin. Topical niacinamide has the potential to reduce the appearance of fine lines and wrinkles, reduce hyperpigmentation spots, and return some of youthful glow to the skin. It has also shown to improve hydration of skin and conditions such as roscea.

RETINOIDS

Retinoids are a group of active ingredients derived from vitamin A. There are a number of different types of retinoids found in skin care products including retinyl palmitate, retinol and tretinoin (retinoic acid). Retinoic acid is the active form of vitamin A derivatives and other forms including retinol and retinyl palmitate must be converted to retinoic acid before they can deliver any beneficial effects to the skin. Retinoic acid is the form found in prescription vitamin A creams.

Retin A has been shown to increase cellular turnover in the top layer of skin making skin appear brighter and smoother. In sun-damaged skin, collagen formation is decreased. Retinoic acid can boost the production of collagen by up to 80 percent and help to restore some of smoothness and plumpness to the skin. This form of vitamin A has also been shown to improve appearance of hyperpigmented lesions such as liver spots and melasma.

PEPTIDES

A peptide is formed when several amino acids are linked. Some peptides are believed to stimulate the formation of collagen and decrease activity of enzymes that destroy elastin.

This action helps the skin to hold some of its resilience. One such peptide is palmitoyl pentapeptide. In test tube studies, this peptide was found to stimulate the formation of collagen, elastin and GAGS. Other peptides, known as neuropeptides, have shown in laboratory results to block the release of neurotransmitters from the nerve to the muscle. One hexapeptide is called Argireline. In theory, this peptide would be able to stop contractions of the muscle revealing a more relaxed look, similar to the actions of botulism toxin A. While results may not be as dramatic as botulism toxin A, one study showed a 30 percent reduction in the depth of wrinkles.

USING YOUR DIET TO SUPPORT HEALTHY SKIN

Healthy skin also starts from the inside. Here are some foods to add to your diet to support a glowing complexion. Mix them in your favorite recipes or eat raw.

1. Garlic and Other High Sulfur Foods

A study published in the *Journal of Nutrition* showed a significant decrease in the production of collagen in the skin of rats fed a low sulfate diet compared to rats fed a diet higher in sulfates. Collagen plays an important role in maintaining the integrity and strength of the skin and gives a younger, more youthful appearance. While there is a paucity of studies directly linking eating foods higher in sulfur with younger looking skin, it would make sense to provide the skin with the basic building blocks it needs to stay strong and supple. Onions, chives, egg yolks and asparagus are rich in sulfur. Proteins such as chicken, fish and legumes are also a good source.

2. Soy Products

Cheese, soy milk and other products made from soy contain genistein – a powerful antioxidant that helps in the production of collagen and slows down the aging of skin. If you wish to keep aging skin at bay, try including some fermented soy products in your diet. One study suggests that genistein may even help speed up wound healing. When applied topically, it has been shown to prevent damage and aging to the skin caused by excessive exposure to sunlight or UV radiation.

3. Foods Rich in Omega-3

Omega-3 is a fatty acid that is considered a "good" fat. Unfortunately, a lot of people do not get enough Omega-3's in their diet. These essential fatty acids promote smooth, supple and soft skin so it is important to take at least 1,000 mg daily. Omega-3 fats are found in most cold-water fish like tuna, salmon and mackerel. If you don't eat fish, you can sprinkle ground flax seeds in your meals, take Omega-3 supplements or flax seed oils. Omega-3 has also shown to minimize the damage in the skin caused by exposure to UV radiation.

4. Red Fruits and Vegetables

Aside from tomatoes, red fruits and vegetables are considered good sources of lycopene and beta carotene. Beets, watermelons and red peppers make tasty additions to your diet. Lycopene and beta carotene have shown to protect the skin from the damage caused by exposure to the sun's ultraviolet rays. This can go a long way in preventing premature aging of the skin.

5. Grapeseed Extract

Derived from the small seeds of red grapes, grapeseed extract is rich in flavonoids and phytochemicals, two compounds packed with antioxidant properties. Grapeseed extract is known to prevent heart disease, fight different types of cancer, skin disease, macular degeneration, cataracts, high cholesterol, as well as fight anti-aging.

Grapeseed extract is proven to enhance skin smoothness and elasticity, as well as fight against free radicals, which are the main culprits in the visual signs of aging. The skin and seeds of grapes are rich in proanthocyanidins, a class of flavonoids commonly found in juice and red wine. Grapeseed can be found in many supplemental forms as well as skin care anti-aging products that are developed exclusively to take advantage of the benefits of the compound.

6. Exercise Nourishes the Skin

We all know that exercise is good for the body, including the heart and lungs and provides a better mental outlook, but regular exercise is also the key to healthy skin. Anything that promotes healthy circulation will also help keep your skin healthy and vibrant. Exercise helps increase blood flow to the skin nourishing cells and keeping them vital.

Blood carries oxygen and nutrients to working cells throughout the body, including the skin. The increased blood flow helps carry waste products, including free radicals from working cells. Exercise does not detoxify the skin – that is the job of the liver.

SKIN – EXFOLIATION
Exfoliation means to remove dead skin cells. There is a basic four-step process to keep your skin glowing and healthy each and every day.

Step 1: Cleansing

Keep it simple. Avoid bar soap because it tends to dry out the skin. Using cleansers that are hypoallergenic and non-comedogenic (do not block pores) may be helpful for all skin types. If you have very dry skin, look for a hydrating cleanser. It is important to cleanse your skin at night before bed to remove all traces of make-up and dirt. Cleanser in the morning may be important as well to remove cells that may have sloughed off overnight and remove any excess sebum production. Never wash your face with hot or cold water as both can cause broken capillaries.

Step 2: Exfoliate

Exfoliating the skin is probably the one step many people skip during their weekly skincare routine. There are several ways to exfoliate the skin:

- **Microdermabrasion or Gentle Facial Scrubs** work by removing the top layer of dead skin cells that tend to dull your complexion. Make sure you use a gentle scrub with tiny grains. Larger grains can be too rough and leave tiny tears in the skin.
- **Chemical Peels** are another way to remove the top layer of skin. There are different grades of chemical peels so it's best to discuss the right one with your skin care physician. Over the counter products that act as chemical peels are labeled with ingredients like glycolic acid, lactic acid and salicylic acid. They usually contain a lower percentage of these ingredients than professional grade products. Even so, an individual with sensitive skin may experience irritation and a

stinging sensation from using these products. Again, if

you are unsure, consult your skin care professional.

- **Retin-A,** or the more moisturizing Renova, removes the top layer of dead skin cells while generating collagen in the skin.

STEP 3: Use a Toner

Toners are meant to remove remaining traces of oil, make-up and dirt, but a good cleanser should do that. Many beauty experts do not use them, but it is totally up to you. If you like the way your skin feels after a toner, then by all means, use a mild one.

Step 4: Moisturize

No matter the skin type, everyone could benefit from a good moisturizer. Choose your moisturizer based on your skin type. Lighter serums may be a better choice for oiler skin types while hydrating creams would be a better choice for dry skin, especially in the winter months. Again seeking out non-comedogenic formulas may help to avoid problems with breakouts and irritation. You can combine a moisturizer with sunscreen to eliminate one step.

What about eye creams? The skin around the eye is thinner and susceptible to fine lines and wrinkles. Another issue is the dreaded dark circles under the eye that can make us appear more tired and older than we are. Many people assume that the circles are caused by a lack of sleep, but there are multiple causes for these bothersome circles. As we age, the skin under the eyes becomes thinner, we lose fatty tissues, and collagen formation slows down. This allows the blood vessels under the skin to become more visible, giving the appearance of dark circles. Those who suffer from allergies and nasal congestion are more prone to dark circles. Lifestyle habits such as smoking, excessive alcohol use, and prolonged excessive stress can also affect the quality and appearance of our skin.

So what can you do? Here are some simple modifications you can do:

- Get a good night sleep – at least 7-8 hours each night. Sleep on your back to minimize repetitive creasing of your face. If you suffer from allergies and/or nasal congestion, consider a purifier in the bedroom, or saline nasal washes (either with a nettie pot or over the counter saline irrigation kit).
- Cool compresses on the eyes may help constrict dilated blood vessel and lessen the appearance of dark circles.
- Wear sunglasses and sunscreen. This protects the eyes, reduces squinting that may exacerbate wrinkle formation, and may reduce excess pigment formation that could make dark circles appear.
- If you are looking for an effective eye cream, one study published in *Journal of Cosmetic Dermatology* showed a combination of vitamin K, vitamin C and vitamin E improved the appearance of under eye circles and showed some improvement in reducing fine lines.

Visit your dermatologist for a complete skin check-up especially if you live in areas with strong sunlight, like Florida or other Southern states. According to the CDC, skin cancer is the most common form of cancer and thousands of people will be diagnosed with melanoma this year. If you develop a new mole or lesion or if there is a change in the appearance of an existing mole, visit your dermatologist promptly. Early detection is a very important part of the treatment of skin cancer.

But what do you do if your skin has already suffered some significant signs of damage and needs a bit more help than topical therapy? Well, the good news is that today's technology provides many other options designed to help enhance collagen production, replace loss volume, minimize lines and wrinkles, and reduce hyperpigmentation spots (age spots).

For example, botulism toxin A can be used to minimize lines and wrinkles around the eyes and forehead, especially those lines that are more pronounced with movement. Fillers such as hyaluronic acid (the same substance present in younger skin) can be used to fill moderate to deep lines and wrinkles around the nose and mouth. Laser technology can be used to treat lines already present in the skin, discolorations, and treat acne and scars. All of these are non-surgical, minimally invasive techniques will not achieve the dramatic after cosmetic surgery, but they can certainly help us to put our best face forward.

**

UPDATE:

Kate's age, habitual facial expression and poor diet had left her with lackluster skin, prominent frown lines between her eyes, and some hyperpigmentation spots on the face. Kate's skin was dry and she was beginning to lose some volume in the face. Her skin care regime called for more hydration, continued nutritional changes to her diet, and a skin care routine targeted to her skin type. A mild retinol product was used at night and a topical vitamin C in the day with a moisturizing sunscreen. For the frown lines between brows that made her look "angry all the time," we injected botulism toxin A, or Botox ®. We also give her a prescription to laugh more and frown less. The results returned the glow to Kate's skin, and revealed a fresh, relaxed appearance.

Closing
Finding Your Center

When we wake up in the morning, we think about preparing our bodies for the day ahead. We may enjoy our morning coffee or tea, take a shower, get dressed, and eat a healthy breakfast. Yet we rarely take the time to prepare our mind and spirit for the day. This doesn't need to take a long time–just a minute or two each morning. A simple morning meditation or prayer can literally transform the way we think, feel, behave, and work.

It helps remind us how blessed we are—even on those days when you sleep through the alarm, when the coffee spills on your lap, when the toast burns, when the kids are whining, when nothing seems to be going right. Before you race out the door, take a moment to take a few deep breaths and focus on your hopes for the new day. Don't forget to take note of something you are thankful for each and every day. You may find that this mediation time is the best part of your day.

Finding Your Center

Within each person, there is a place that holds the essence of who you really are–your center. It is not a physical place, but rather a place of certainty and confidence. When you are stressed, it is good to contemplate this place so you can reconnect with calm certainty.

So "finding your center" means understanding that any stressful situation or circumstance you are dealing with will pass. You will learn from it and remain calm and focused. This is important when events make you crazy. When your world falls apart, your center reassures you that the event will pass, but you will remain the same person. Your center is a place of calm; a place within you that provides great strength and resolve. It is the place to refresh and renew.

One of my favorite sayings sums up finding your space: *If you are in emotional distress, "finding your center" can remind you that you are stronger than you realize, and that you need to reconnect with your essential being.*

Have you ever been swimming in a lake or the ocean and dove down deep enough where it felt so quiet and peaceful, but you knew that on the surface of the water above, there were waves, wind and chaos? This metaphor can be used in our own lives when facing illness, disease or relationship problems. The peacefulness of floating under water illustrates life's challenges and difficult times. Sometimes it feels like there is a storm swirling around us with very few breaks to regroup. It is during these most challenging times when we need to connect to our wiser, inner self. However, accessing this place of calm and remembering it on a daily basis may require some practice, especially in the midst of chaos.

Change takes place in our lives constantly making us feel edgy, fearful, and certainly not peaceful. It is that constant state of flux that makes it difficult to find your center and feel grounded. We may be going through difficult times in our business, marriage, or other relationships, and sometimes we need some time to feel grounded again.

Referring back to the water metaphor (or another peaceful image you may have) gives us the opportunity to look at life from a different perspective. Taking the time to write down our thoughts helps us to make clear and focused decisions that are not driven by emotion. Here are some ways to apply this process to your own life.

Step 1: Recognize the space you're presently in. Are things feeling out of control? Is it difficult to make decisions? Do you feel a lack of energy, have trouble sleeping even though you're exhausted, and a general feeling of discontent? Can you pinpoint exactly what is nagging you? Once you have a sense of the problem, it is easier to do something about it.

Step 2: If you've ever done any personal development work, go back to a structure that worked for you. It might be listening to your favorite music, talking to a friend, or writing in a journal. Choose a method that works for you and spend some time remembering what's important and what makes you feel good. Another great exercise to do is to write down 10 things you're grateful or proud of. Shifting your energy to what works rather than focusing on what doesn't work will serve you more.

Step 3: Make a list of your options. What choices do you have? Even if you feel you don't have any choices, you do! This is like a big brainstorming session and it's important to allow every possible choice to surface, even the ones that seem ridiculous or absurd.

Step 4: If you didn't do so in the step above, look at each choice again and consider the possible outcomes for each option. Literally try on that choice – stand up, move to another space and "try it on." How does it feel? What do you imagine will happen? What are all of the scenarios? Write down any insights you have. Say each choice aloud and pay attention to your body. Find one that resonates or make you feel the most "alive."

Step 5: Now take some action – any action. Notice the fear you feel even reading that statement. It's OK to feel afraid. Remember courage is acting in spite of your fear. Do something – anything - and see what happens.

Having dreams can also help you overcome difficult circumstances in your life. Even though they may or may not come true, they make it possible to get through the challenges in life with determination and a sense of hope. Find your passion and purpose in life and do what you love to do. Find others that share the same passion as you do.

Accepting Ourselves

The first fundamental step to "centering" is self-acceptance. We are who we are and we need to make the most of it, instead of envying others for their possessions, their appearance or their lifestyle. Stop comparing yourself to others and encourage yourself to reach your highest potential. Self-acceptance will come progressively as you try to live up to the highest standard that is right for you.

Kindness

Acceptance leads to the second attitude necessary for finding your own center: kindness. It is difficult to connect to that place of calm when you find yourself obsessing about your shortcomings or hating yourself. Practicing kindness starts with you. Practicing kindness means acknowledging that you will not be the master of everything, and at the same time giving yourself permission to improve things you need or want. Extend this kindness and non-judgment to others. Remember that your path is not the only path and it can go a long way towards helping you to maintain your center.

A Process of Unlearning

Finding your center is not a process of divorcing yourself from objective reality, but rather reaching a universal center. This process of "unlearning" and "relearning" allows you to rise above the usual level of understanding gleaned from superficial facts and observations.

Wisdom gained from tuning in to your own center is similar to going to school, where the goal is to learn. Meditation is a simply a process of unlearning. This doesn't mean that we should try to forget all the knowledge we acquired in school or in life. That knowledge has its own place and purpose. Instead, meditation and other modalities used to quiet the mind and external chatter can be used to greatly sharpen the intellect. What we must "unlearn" are the delusions of limitations imposed by our own egos.

Let go of everything that's unhealthy, stressful or ineffective. This may be a relationship, food, or a lifestyle choice that no longer works for you. We have already discussed the healing properties of healthy, supportive relationships, healthy lifestyle and food choices, and effective stress management. However, what if the problem is holding too tightly to an idea of how we think something should work? For example, what if we develop tunnel vision about what we think it means to be healthy? This narrow vision can keep us off center and even be potentially dangerous to our health. Remember, the first step to finding your center is to be present now. If something is not working, change it–whatever the situation. If you have a potentially life-threatening infection, treat it with antibiotics. If you have dangerously high blood pressure, realize you may need blood pressure medicine. If you have asthma and you can't breathe, use your inhaler. It is what you do that matters. In my opinion, living naturally means living responsibly. Find out what you can do to take charge of your health. Trading pharmaceutical medicines for herbal medicines does not bring about balance.

Both can be potentially healing or harmful depending how they are used.

Balance is acknowledging and taking advantage of the interconnection between the body, mind and spirit.

Treat acute issues by using the most effective treatment with the least side effects for you, and then go a step further. Look at the areas in your life that may be contributing to the process. Do you need to make a lifestyle, nutritional, mental, social, or an environmental change? Can you access the part of your being that allows you to do your best and then let go? By looking at all of these aspects of your life, you can chart a path to optimal wellness.

APPENDIX

TABLE 9: ORAC

http://www.ars.usda.gov/is/pr/1999/990208.htm

GROCERY LIST: Here is a detailed listing of healthy proteins, vegetables and fruits that you should consume each day for a healthy, balanced diet.

Grocery Shopping List

PROTEIN SOURCES

Eggs or egg whites
Egg whites
Fish – salmon, tuna, halibut, cod, orange roughy, tilapia
Shellfish – (limit to 1 to 2 times per week)
Chicken or turkey breast
Lean beef – buffalo, venison, lamb
Tofu
Tempeh

LEGUMES
1 to 2 servings per day
Servings size = ½ cup, cooked

Beans – garbanzo, pinto, fat-free refried, black, lima, cannellini, navy, mung, hummus (1/4 cup)
Edamame (green soybeans)
Peas – yellow and green split peas, sweet green peas
Lentils – red and green
Bean soups

LOW GLYCEMIC VEGETABLES

Consume unlimited servings per day. Eat fresh, frozen or organic when possible. Avoid canned vegetables.

Asparagus
Artichokes
Bean Sprouts
Bell Peppers
Broccoli
Brussels Sprouts
Cauliflower
Celery
Cucumber
Cabbage family – red, green, Chinese
Onions family – chives, leeks, garlic
Green Beans
Mushrooms
Okra
Radishes
Snow peas
Sprouts
Salsa – no sugar added
Tomatoes
Water chestnuts – 5 whole
Squash – zucchini, yellow or spaghetti
Kelps – all types – dulce, wakame, nori
Leafy Greens – bok choy, escarole, spinach, dandelion, mustard, beet
Mixed Greens - romaine, red and green leaf, endive, arugula, radicchio, watercress, chicory

HIGH GLYCEMIC VEGETABLES

Limit to one serving per day and consume with a protein source

Serving size = ½ cup or as specified

Beets

Carrots = raw = 2 whole or 12 baby

Winter squash – acorn, butternut, pumpkin

Potatoes – sweet potatoes, yams, russet, white or red

FATS and OILS

Four servings per day

Serving size = 1 teaspoon

Oils should cold pressed

Flaxseed – refrigerate

Walnut oil

Extra virgin olive oil

Canola oil

Sesame oil

Olives – ripe or green, limit to eight

Avocado - ¼ of a whole one

Mayonnaise made with canola or flax oil

Butter – limit to one teaspoon per day

NUTS and SEEDS

Servings per day = 2

Almonds – whole – 10 to 15 nuts

Hazelnuts – 10 to 15 nuts

Natural nut butters – 1 tablespoon

Peanuts – 9 to 12 nuts

Sunflower seeds – 2 tablespoons

Pumpkin seeds – 2 tablespoons

Sesame seeds –2 tablespoons

WHOLE GRAINS (avoid wheat or gluten if intolerant)
Two servings per day
Serving Size = ½ cup

Amaranth
Teff
Quinoa
Rice – basmati, brown, wild
Corn tortillas- no more than 2
Pasta – preferably made from rice or corn instead of wheat; limit to 2 to 3 servings per week
Breads – 1 slice, made from rice or gluten-free
Crackers – 3 crackers, gluten-free
Cereals – ½ cup, free from gluten, wheat and dairy

FRUIT
1 to 2 servings per day

Apple – 1 medium
Apricot – 1 medium
Blackberries – ½ cup
Blueberries – ½ cup
Raspberries – 1 cup
Strawberries – 1 cup
Cherries – ½ cup
Grapes – ½ cup
Melon – ½ Cantaloupe, ¼ Honeydew
Nectarine – 2 small
Peach – 2 small
Kiwi – 2 small
Tangerine – 2 small
Plum – 3 small
Mango
Papaya

BEVERAGES

Coffee – (minus sugars and creams)- limit to 2 cups daily

Teas

Purified Water

Mineral Water – plain or flavored unsweetened

REFERENCES:

Leander K, Hallqvist J., Reuterwall C., et al Family History of Coronary Heart Disease, a Strong Risk Factor for Myocardial Infarction Interacting with Other Cardiovascular Risk Factors: Results from the Stockholm Heart Epidemiology Program (SHEEP) *Epidemiology* 2001; 12:215-221.

S. Pohjola-Sintonen, A. Rissanen, P. Liskola, and K. Luomanmäki. Family history as a risk factor of coronary heart disease in patients under 60 years of age. *Eur Heart J* 1998; 19: 235-239.

W. Bao, S.R. Srinivasan, R. Valdez. Longitudinal Changes in Cardiovascular Risk From Childhood to Young Adulthood in Offspring of Parents With Coronary Artery Disease. *JAMA*. 1997;278(21):1749-1754.

R.E Vlietstra; R.A. Kronmal; A. Oberman; et al. Effect of Cigarette Smoking on Survival of Patients With Angiographically Documented Coronary Artery Disease. *JAMA*. 1986;255(8):1023-1027.

Sessa WC, Pritchard K, Seyedi N, Wang J and Hintze TH. Chronic exercise in dogs increases coronary vascular nitric oxide production and endothelial cell nitric oxide synthase gene expression. *Circulation Research*. 1994; 74: 349-353.

Narayan KM, Boyle JP, Thompson TJ, Sorensen SW, Williamson DF. "Lifetime risk for diabetes mellitus in the United States". *JAMA* 2003. 290 (14): 1884–90.

Maahs DM., Hamman RF., D'Agostino R., et al. The Association between Adiponectin/Leptin Ratio and Diabetes. *Journal of Pediatrics* 2009;155(1):133-135.

Haney EM, Chan BK, Diem SJ, Ensrud KE, Cauley JA, et al. Association of low bone mineral density with selective serotonin reuptake inhibitor use by older men. *Arch Intern Med.* 2007;167(12):1246-51.

Raffaele N, Vincenzo G, Valentina A, et al. Acute Effects of Triiodothyronine on Endothelial Function in Human Subjects. *The Journal of Clinical Endocrinology & Metabolism.* 2007; 92(1): 250-254.

Dyke CM, Ding M, Abd-Elfattah AS, et al. Effects of triiodothyronine supplementation after myocardial ischemia. *Ann Thorac Surg.* 1993: 56(2):215-22.

Danforth E Jr, Burger A. The role of thyroid hormones in the control of energy expenditure. *Clin Endocrinol Metab.* 1984;13(3):581-95.

Klemperer JD, Zelano J, Helm RE, et al. Triiodothyronine improves left ventricular function without oxygen wasting effects after global hypothermic ischemia. *J Thorac Cardiovasc Surg.* 1995;109(3):457-65.

Robertas B, Gintautas K, Rimas Ž, and Prange Jr. A. Effects of Thyroxine as Compared with Thyroxine Plus Triiodothyronine in Patients with Hypothyroidism. *N Engl J Med* 1999; 340:424-429.

Kralik A, Eder K, Kirchgessner M. Influence of zinc and selenium deficiency on parameters relating to thyroid hormone metabolism. *Horm Metab Res.* 1996;28(5):223-6.

Davis, S, Moreau, M, Kroll, R, et al. for the APHRODITE Study Team.
Testosterone for Low Libido in Postmenopausal Women Not Taking Estrogen.
N Engl J Med 2008; 359:2005-2017.

Lemon, H, Wotiz, H, Parsons, L, et al. Reduced Estriol Excretion in Patients With Breast Cancer Prior to Endocrine Therapy. *JAMA*. 1966;196(13):1128-1136.

Lippman, M, Monaco, M, Bolan, G. Effects of Estrone, Estradiol, and Estriol on Hormone-responsive Human Breast Cancer in Long-Term Tissue Culture. *Cancer Res.* June 1977 *37;* 1901.

Coelingh B, Singer C, Simoncini T, et al. Estetrol, a pregnancy-specific human steroid, prevents and suppresses mammary tumor growth in a rat model. *Climacteric 11* 2008: (Suppl 1) 29.

Coelingh B, Skouby, P, Bouchard, C.F., et al. Ovulation inhibition by estetrol in an in vivo model. *Climacteric 11: 2008.* (Suppl 1). 30 (a summary from *Contraception* 77(3) (2008) 186-190).

Holinka, C.F, Brincat, M, Coelingh B. Preventive effect of oral estetrol in a menopausal hot flush model. *Climacteric 11*: 2008 (Suppl 1) 15-21.

Coelingh B, Heegaard, AM, Visser, M. et al. Oral bioavailability and bone-sparing effects of estetrol in an osteoporosis model. *Climacteric 11*: 2008. (Suppl 1) 2-14.

Sex hormones influence on the immune system: basic and clinical aspects in autoimmunity. *Lupus.* 2004; 13(9): 635-638.

Pentikäinen V, Erkkilä K, Suomalainen, L, Parvinen M, Dunkel L. Estradiol acts as a germ cell survival factor in the human testis in vitro. *The Journal of Clinical Endocrinology and Metabolism* 2000; 85 (5): 2057–67.

Lasiuk GC, Hegadoren KM. The effects of estradiol on central serotonergic systems and its relationship to mood in women. *Biol Res Nurs.* 2007; 9 (2): 147–60.

Carreau S, Lambard S, Delalande C, Denis-Galeraud I, Bourguiba S,. Aromatase expression and role of estrogens in male gonad: a review. *Reproductive Biology and Endocrinology* 2003; 1: 35.

Bonkhoff, H, Fixemer, T, Hunsicker, I, Remberger, K. Estrogen receptor expression in prostate cancer and premalignant prostatic lesions. *Am J Pathol.* 1999;155(2):641-7.

Emmelot-Vonk MH, et al. Effect of testosterone supplementation on functional mobility, cognition, and other parameters in older men: A randomized controlled trial. *JAMA.* 2008;299:39.

Amore M, et al. Partial androgen deficiency, depression and testosterone treatment in aging men. *Aging Clinical and Experimental Research* 2009;21:1.

Kingsberg S, Shifren J, Wekselman K, Rodenberg C, Koochaki P, Derogatis L. Evaluation of the clinical relevance of benefits associated with transdermal testosterone treatment in postmenopausal women with hypoactive sexual desire disorder. *J Sex Med.* 2007;4(4 Pt 1):1001-8.

Simon J, Braunstein G, Nachtigall L, Utian W, Katz M, Miller S, et al. Testosterone patch increases sexual activity and desire in surgically menopausal women with hypoactive sexual desire disorder. *J Clin Endocrinol Metab.* 2005;90(9):5226-33; *Epub* 2005 Jul 12.

Raman, JD; Schlegel, PN. Aromatase inhibitors for male infertility. *The Journal of Urology. 2002;*167 (2 Pt 1): 624–9

Sharpe, RM; Skakkebaek, NE. Are estrogens involved in falling sperm counts and disorders of the male reproductive tract? *Lancet. 1993;* 341 (8857): 1392–5.

Wright D, Kellermann A, Hertzberg V, et al. ProTECT: A Randomized Clinical Trial of Progesterone for Acute Traumatic Brain Injury *Annals of Emergency Medicine.* Volume 49, Issue 4, pages 391-402.e2.

Foidart JM, Colin C, Denoo X, Desreux J, Béliard A, Fournier S, De Lignières B.
Estradiol and progesterone regulate the proliferation of human breast epithelial cells. *Fertility and Sterility.* 1998; 69 (5): 963-969.

Harris B, Lovett L, Newcombe RG, Read GF, Walker R, Riad-Fahmy D. Maternity blues and major endocrine changes: Cardiff puerperal mood and hormone study *IIBMJ.* 1994;308:949.

Sarkola T, Mäkisalo H, Fukunaga T, Eriksson P. Acute Effect of Alcohol on Estradiol, Estrone, Progesterone, Prolactin, Cortisol, and Luteinizing Hormone in Premenopausal Women. *Alcoholism: Clinical and Experimental Research.* 1999; 23 (6): 976–982.

Christen Y. Oxidative stress and Alzheimer's Disease. *Am J Clin Nutr.* 2000; 71(2):621S-629S.

Diaz M, Frei B, Vita J, Keaney Jr, J. Antioxidants and Atherosclerotic Heart Disease *N Engl J Med.* 1997; 337:408-416.

Vita J, Keaney Jr J, Raby K, et al. Low Plasma Ascorbic Acid Independently Predicts the Presence of an Unstable Coronary Syndrome. *Journal of the American College of Cardiology.* 1998; 31(5): 980–986.

Halvorsen B, Carlsen M, Phillips K, et al. Content of redox-active compounds (ie. antioxidants) in foods consumed in the United States. *American Journal of Clinical Nutrition.* 2006; 84(1): 95-135.

Carr A, Zhu B, Frei B. Potential Antiatherogenic Mechanisms of Ascorbate (Vitamin C) and α-Tocopherol (Vitamin E). *Circulation Research.* 2000;87:349-354.

Zhu Y, Xia M, Yang Y, et al. Purified Anthocyanin Supplementation Improves Endothelial Function via NO-cGMP Activation in Hypercholesterolemic Individuals. *Clin Chem.* 2011;57(11):1524-33. *Epub* 2011 Sep 16.

Mauray A, Felgines C, Morand C, Mazur A, Scalbert A, Milenkovic D. Nutrigenomic analysis of the protective effects of bilberry anthocyanin-rich extract in apo E-deficient mice. *Genes Nutr.* 2010;5(4):343-53. *Epub* 2010 Mar 1.

Prior RL, Wu X, Gu L, Hager T, Hager A, Wilkes S, et al. Purified berry anthocyanins but not whole berries normalize lipid parameters in mice fed an obesogenic high fat diet. *Mol Nutr Food Res.* 2009;53(11):1406-18.

Vaccinium macrocarpon: an interesting option for women with recurrent urinary tract infections and other health benefits. *J Obstet Gynaecol Res.* 2009;35(4):630-9.

Ahuja S, Kaack B, Roberts J. Loss of fimbrial adhesion with the addition of vaccinum macrocarpon to the growth medium of P-fimbriated Escherichia coli. *J Urol.* 1998;159:559-562.

Burger O, Ofek I, Tabak M, et al. A high molecular mass constituent of cranberry juice inhibits helicobacter pylori adhesion to human gastric mucus. *FEMS Immunol Med Microbiol.* 2000;29(4):295-301.

Kim MJ, Ohn J, Kim JH, Kwak HK. Effects of freeze-dried cranberry powder on serum lipids and inflammatory markers in lipopolysaccharide treated rats fed an atherogenic diet. *Nutr Res Pract.* 2011; 5(5):404-11. Epub 2011 Oct 28.

Chen W, Rosner B, Hankinson S, Colditz G, Willett W. Moderate Alcohol Consumption During Adult Life, Drinking Patterns, and Breast Cancer Risk. *JAMA.* 2011;306(17):1884-1890.

Alcohol attributable burden of incidence of cancer in eight European countries based on results from prospective cohort study. *BMJ.* 2011;342:d1584.

U.S. Department of Health and Human Services. The Health Consequences of Smoking: A Report of the Surgeon General. U.S. Department of Health and Human Services, Centers for Disease Control and Prevention, National Center for Chronic Disease Prevention and Health Promotion, Office on Smoking and Health, 2004.

Phase II Study of Pomegranate Juice for Men with Rising Prostate-Specific Antigen following Surgery or Radiation for Prostate Cancer. *Clin Cancer Res*. July 1, 2006 *12;* 4018.

Aviram M, Dornfeld L. Pomegranate juice consumption inhibits serum angiotensin converting enzyme activity and reduces systolic blood pressure. *Atherosclerosis*. 2001;158(1):195-8.

Aviram M, Rosenblat M, Gaitini D, et al. Pomegranate juice consumption for 3 years by patients with carotid artery stenosis reduces common carotid intima-media thickness, blood pressure and LDL oxidation. *Clin Nutr*. 2004;23(3):423-433.

Khan GN, Gorin MA, Rosenthal D, Pan Q, et al. Pomegranate fruit extract impairs invasion and motility in human breast cancer. *Integr Cancer Ther*. 2009;8(3):242-53.

Hadipour-Jahromy M, Mozaffari-Kermani R. Chondroprotective effects of pomegranate juice on monoiodoacetate-induced osteoarthritis of the knee joint of mice. *Phytother Res*. 2009 Jun 5.

Effects of dietary coconut oil on the biochemical and anthropometric profiles of women presenting abdominal obesity. *Lipids*. 2009.

The cholesterol-lowering effect of coconut flakes in humans with moderately raised serum cholesterol. *J Med Food*. 2004.

Rettig MB, Heber D, An J, Seeram NP, Rao JY, et al. Pomegranate extract inhibits androgen-independent prostate cancer growth through a nuclear factor-kappaB-dependent mechanism. *Mol Cancer Ther*. 2008;7(9):2662-71. Erratum in: *Mol Cancer Ther*. 2008;7(11):3654.

Sartippour MR, Seeram NP, Rao JY, Moro A, Harris DM, et al. Ellagitannin-rich pomegranate extract inhibits angiogenesis in prostate cancer in vitro and in vivo. *Int J Oncol.* 2008;32(2):475-80.

Giovannucci E, Rimm E, Liu Y, Stampfer M, Willett W. A Prospective Study of Tomato Products, Lycopene, and Prostate Cancer Risk. *JNCI J Natl Cancer Inst.* 2002:94(5): 391-398. doi: 10.1093/jnci/94.5.391.

Milner JA. Garlic: Its anticarcinogenic and antitumorigenic properties. *Nutrition Reviews.* 1996; 54:S82–S86.

Pinto J, Rivlin R. Antiproliferative Effects of Allium Derivatives from Garlic. *J. Nutr.* 2001;131 (3): 1058S-1060S.

Kambara T, McFarlane RG, Abell TJ, McAnulty RW, Sykes AR. The effect of age and dietary protein on immunity and resistance in lambs vaccinated with Trichostrongylus colubriformis. *International Journal for Parasitology.* 1993; 23 (4):471–476.

Daly JM, Reynolds J, Sigal RK, Shou J, Liberman MD. Department of Surgery, University of Pennsylvania School of Medicine, Philadelphia. Effect of dietary protein and amino acids on immune function. *Crit Care Med.* 1990;18(2 Suppl):S86-93.

Engler MM. Comparative study of diets enriched with evening primrose, black currant, borage or fungal oils on blood pressure and pressor responses in spontaneously hypertensive rats. *Prostaglandins Leukot Essent Fatty Acids.* 1993;49(4): 809-14.

Mozaffarian D, Ascherio A, Hu FB, et al. Interplay between different polyunsaturated fatty acids and risk of coronary heart disease in men. *Circulation.* 2005;111(2):157-164.

Von Schacky C. The role of omega-3 fatty acids in cardiovascular disease. *Curr. Atheroscler. Rep.* 2003;**5** (2):139–45.

Gerster H. Can adults adequately convert alpha-linolenic acid (18:3n-3) to eicosapentaenoic acid (20:5n-3) and docosahexaenoic acid (22:6n-3)? *Int. J. Vitam. Nutr. Res.* 1998: 68 (3):159–173.

Brenna JT. Efficiency of conversion of alpha-linolenic acid to long chain n-3 fatty acids in man. *Curr. Opin. Clin. Nutr. Metab. Care.* 2002; 5 (2):127–132.

Hu FB, Stampfer MJ, Manson JE, et al. Dietary intake of alpha-linolenic acid and risk of fatal ischemic heart disease among women. *Am J Clin Nutr.* 1999;69(5):890-897.

Rallidis LS, Paschos G, Liakos GK, Velissaridou AH, Anastasiadis G, Zampelas A. Dietary alpha-linolenic acid decreases C-reactive protein, serum amyloid A and interleukin-6 in dyslipidaemic patients. *Atherosclerosis.* 2003;167(2):237-242.

From the Jean Mayer USDA Human Nutrition Research Center on Aging at Tufts University, Boston. Effect of dietary supplementation with black currant seed oil on the immune response of healthy elderly subjects. *American Journal of Clinical Nutrition.* 1999: 70(4): 536-543.

Villegas R, et al. The cumulative effect of core lifestyle behaviours on the prevalence of hypertension and dyslipidemia. *BMC Public Health.* 2008;8:210.

Your guide to lowering blood pressure with DASH. National Heart, Lung, and Blood Institute. ttp://www.nhlbi.nih.gov/health/public/heart/hbp/dash/new_das h.pdf. Accessed June 8, 2010.

Appel LJ, et al. Dietary approaches to prevent and treat hypertension: A scientific statement from the American Heart Association. *Hypertension*. 2006;47:296.

Guerrero-Romero F, Rodríguez-Morán M. The effect of lowering blood pressure by magnesium supplementation in diabetic hypertensive adults with low serum magnesium levels: a randomized, double-blind, placebo-controlled clinical trial. *J Hum Hypertens*. 2009;23(4):245-51.

Villegas R, et al. The cumulative effect of core lifestyle behaviours on the prevalence of hypertension and dyslipidemia. *BMC Public Health*. 2008;8:210.

Li Y, Zhang T, Korkaya H, Liu S, Lee HF, Newman B, et al. Department of Pharmaceutical Sciences, College of Pharmacy, University of Michigan. Sulforaphane, a dietary component of broccoli/broccoli sprouts, inhibits breast cancer stem cells. *Clin Cancer Res*. 2010; 1;16(9):2580-90. Epub 2010 Apr 13.

Abdulah R, Faried A, Kobayashi K, Yamazaki C, Suradji EW, Ito K, et al. Department of Public Health, Gunma University Graduate School of Medicine, Japan. Selenium enrichment of broccoli sprout extract increases chemosensitivity and apoptosis of LNCaP prostate cancer cells. *BMC Cancer*. 2009 Nov 30;9:414.

Elisa Bandera, one of the authors of the American Cancer Society's 2006 Guidelines on Nutrition and Physical Activity for Cancer Prevention. The 42-page report published in the

September/October 2006 issue of *CA: a Cancer Journal for Clinicians.*

Riserus U, Willett WC, Hu FB. Dietary fats and prevention of Type 2 diabetes. *Prog Lipid Res.* 2009;48:44-51.

Fung TT, Rexrode KM, Mantzoros CS, Manson JE, Willett WC, Hu FB. Mediterranean diet and incidence of and mortality from coronary heart disease and stroke in women. *Circulation.* 2009;119:1093-100.

Kastorini CM, Milionis HJ, Esposito K, Giugliano D, Goudevenos JA, Panagiotakos DB. The effect of Mediterranean diet on metabolic syndrome and its components: a meta-analysis of 50 studies and 534,906 individuals. *J Am Coll Cardiol.* 2011;57:1299-313.

C-Reactive Protein, a Sensitive Marker of Inflammation, Predicts Future Risk of Coronary Heart Disease in Initially Healthy Middle-Aged Men. *Circulation.* 1999;99:237-242.

Ndumele CE, Pradhan AD, Ridker PM. Department of Medicine, Brigham and Women's Hospital, Harvard Medical School, Boston, MA. Interrelationships between inflammation, C-reactive protein, and insulin resistance. *J Cardiometab Syndr.* 2006;1(3):190-6.

Libby P, Ridker PM. Brigham and Women's Hospital, Boston, MA. Inflammation and atherosclerosis: role of C-reactive protein in risk assessment. *Am J Med.* 2004;116 Suppl 6A:9S-16S.

Morrison C. Interaction Between Exercise and Leptin in the Treatment of Obesity. *Diabetes.* 2008; 57(3):534-535.

Shapiro A, Matheny M, Zhang Y, Tümer N, Cheng Kit-Yan, Rogrigues E, et al. Synergy Between Leptin Therapy and a Seemingly Negligible Amount of Voluntary Wheel Running Prevents Progression of Dietary Obesity in Leptin-Resistant Rats. *Diabetes*. 2008;57(3):614-622.

Leptin and Insulin Sensitivity, Dissertation, John Joseph Dube, U. Pittsburg, Depts. of Health and Physical Activity and School of Medicine, 2005. http://etd.library.pitt.edu/ETD/available/etd-04112005-095658/unrestricted/dube_etd_2005.pdf

Investigation, Rohit N. Kulkami, M.D., Ph.D, et al: Uncover potential role of leptin in diabetes. *The Journal of Clinical*. October 2007. http://www.joslin.harvard.edu/news/joslin_researchers_uncover_potential_role_of_leptin_in_diabetes.html

Diabetes Prevention Program Research Group; Reduction in the incidence of Type 2 diabetes with lifestyle intervention or metformin. *N Engl J Med*. 2002; 346(6): 393–403.

Herman WH, Hoerger TJ, Brandle M, Hicks K, Sorensen S, Zhang P, et al. Diabetes Prevention Program Research Group. The cost-effectiveness of lifestyle modification or metformin in preventing type 2 diabetes in adults with impaired glucose tolerance. *Ann Intern Med*. 2005;142(5):323-32.

Richards J, Johnson T, Kuzma J, Lonac M, Schweder M, Voyles W, Bell C. Short-term sprint interval training increases insulin sensitivity in healthy adults but does not affect the thermogenic response to β-adrenergic stimulation. *J Physiol*. 2010; 588(Pt 15): 2961–2972.

Arnt Erik Tjønna, MSc; Sang Jun Lee, PhD; Øivind Rognmo, MSc; Tomas O. ølen,MSc; Anja Bye, MSc; Per Magnus Haram, PhD; Jan Pål Loennechen, PhD; Qusai Y. Al-Share, MSc; Eirik Skogvoll, PhD; Stig A. Slørdahl, PhD; Ole J. Kemi, PhD; Sonia M. Najjar, PhD; Ulrik Wisløff, PhD : Aerobic Interval Training Versus Continuous Moderate Exercise as a Treatment for the Metabolic Syndrome. *Circulation.* 2008;118:346-354.

Houmard J, Tanner C, Slentz C, Duscha B, McCartney J, Kraus W. Effect of the volume and intensity of exercise training on insulin sensitivity. *Journal of Applied Physiology.* 2004;96(1):101-106.

Umpierre D, Ribeiro P, Kramer C, Leitão C, Zucatti A, Azevedo M, et al. Physical Activity Advice Only or Structured Exercise Training and Association With HbA$_{1c}$ Levels in Type 2 Diabetes. *JAMA.* 2011;305(17):1790-1799.

Tran ZV, Weltman A, Glass GV, Mood DP. The effects of exercise on blood lipids and lipoproteins: a meta-analysis of studies. *Medicine and Science in Sports and Exercise.* 1983; 15(5):393-402.

Climbing exercise enhances osteoblast differentiation and inhibits adipogenic differentiation with high expression of PTH/PTHrP receptor in bone marrow cells. *Bone.* 2008; 43(3): 613-620.

The effects of muscle-building exercise on forearm bone mineral content and osteoblast activity in drug-free and anabolic steroids self-administering young men. (PMID:2065220). Clinica Medica 2, University of Catania O.V.E, Italy. *Bone and Mineral.* 1991; 13(1):77-83.

Hance, Kenneth W., et al. Combination of physical activity, nutrition, or other metabolic factors and vaccine response. *Front Biosci.* 2007;12:4997–5029.

Woods JA, et al. Exercise and cellular innate immune function. *Med Sci Sports Exerc.* 1999;31(1):57-66.

Oken BS, Zajdel D, Kishiyama S, et al. Randomized, controlled, six-month trial of yoga in healthy seniors: effects on cognition and quality of life. *Alternative Therapies in Health and Medicine.* 2006;12(1):40–47.

Raub, JA. Psychophysiologic effects of hatha yoga on musculoskeletal and cardiopulmonary function: a literature review. *The Journal of Alternative and Complementary Medicine.* 2002;8(6):797–812.

Yang K. A review of yoga programs for four leading risk factors of chronic diseases. *Evidence-Based Complementary and Alternative Medicine.* 2007;4(4):487–491.

Pratley R, Nicklas B, Rubin M, Miller J, Smith A, Smith M, et al. Strength training increases resting metabolic rate and norepinephrine levels in healthy 50- to 65-yr old men. *J Appl Physiol.*
1994;76:133–137.

American College of Sports Medicine position stand: the recommended quantity and quality of exercise for developing and maintaining cardiorespiratory and muscular fitness and flexibility in healthy adults. *Med Sci Sports Exerc.* 1998;30:975–991.

Pate RR, Pratt M, Blair SN, Haskell WL, Macera CA, Bouchard C, et al. Physical activity and public health: a recommendation from the Centers for Disease Control and Prevention and the American College of Sports Medicine. *JAMA.* 1995;273:402–407.

Ades PA, Ballor DL, Ashikaga T, Utton JL, Nair KS. Weight training improves walking endurance in healthy elderly persons. *Ann Intern Med.* 1996;124:568–572.

Hilyer JC, Brown KC, Sirles AT, Peoples L. A flexibility intervention to reduce the incidence and severity of joint injuries among municipal firefighters. *J Occup Med.* 1990;32:631–637.

Beneficial effects of docosahexaenoic acid on cognition in age-related cognitive decline Alzheimer's & Dementia. *The Journal of the Alzheimer's Association.* 2010; 6(6):456-464.

Sapolsky RM, Krey LC, McEwen BS. The adrenocortical stress-response in the aged male rat: impairment of recovery from stress. *Exp Gerontol.* 1983;18(1):55-64.

Sapolsky RM. Department of Biological Sciences, Stanford University, CA. Do glucocorticoid concentrations rise with age in the rat? *Neurobiol Aging.* 1992;13(1):171-4.

Lupien SJ, et al. Cortisol levels during human aging predict hippocampal atrophy and memory deficits. *Nat Neurosci.* 1998;1:69.

Davis LL, Weaver M, Zamrini E, Stevens A, Kang DH, Parker CR Jr. Biopsychological markers of distress in informal caregivers. *Biol Res Nurs.* 2004 Oct;6(2):90-9.

Holmes Rahe Social Readjustment Rating Scale Adult Stress. *Journal of Psychosomatic Research,* 1967, vol. II p. 214.

Ernst, O, Pinel, C. Neuroscience Program, UBC Hospital, University of British Columbia; Olson, Pinel, Christie — Department of Psychology, UBC Hospital, University of British Columbia; Christie — Brain Research Centre, UBC Hospital, University of British Columbia; Lam — Division of Clinical Neuroscience, Department of Psychiatry, University of British Columbia, and Mood Disorders Centre, UBC Hospital, Vancouver, BC; Antidepressant effects of exercise: Evidence for an adult-neurogenesis hypothesis? *J Psychiatry Neurosci.* 2006 March; 31(2): 84–92.

Vallée M, MacCari S, Dellu F, Simon H, Le Moal M, Mayo W. INSERM U.259, Université de Bordeaux II, Domaine de Carreire, France. Long-term effects of prenatal stress and postnatal handling on age-related glucocorticoid secretion and cognitive performance: a longitudinal study in the rat. *Eur J Neurosci.* 1999;11(8):2906-16.

Takahashi LK. Department of Psychiatry, University of Wisconsin Medical School, Madison, WI. Prenatal stress: consequences of glucocorticoids on hippocampal development and function. *Int J Dev Neurosci.* 1998;16(3-4):199-207.

Conrad CD, et al. Chronic stress impairs rat spatial memory on the Y maze, and this effect is blocked by tianeptine pretreatment. *Behav Neurosci.* 1996;110:1321.
Song L, et al. Impairment of the spatial learning and memory induced by learned helplessness and chronic mild stress. *Pharmacol Biochem Behav.* 2006;83:186.

McLay RN, Freeman SM, Zadina JE. Chronic corticosterone impairs memory performance in the Barnes maze. *Physiol Behav.* 1998;63:933.

Egeland J, et al. Cortisol level predicts executive and memory function in depression, symptom level predicts psychomotor speed. *Acta Psychiatr Scand.* 2005;112:434.

Mondelli V, Cattaneo A, Belvederi Murri M, Di Forti M, Handley R, Hepgul N, et al. Stress and inflammation reduce brain-derived neurotrophic factor expression in first-episode psychosis: a pathway to smaller hippocampal volume. *J Clin Psychiatry.* 2011;72(12):1677-84. Epub 2011 May 18.

Marais L, Stein DJ, Daniels WM. Exercise increases BDNF levels in the striatum and decreases depressive-like behavior in chronically stressed rats. *Metab Brain Dis.* 2009;24(4):587-97. Epub 2009 Oct 21.

Wurtman RJ, Wurtman JJ. Do carbohydrates affect food intake via neurotransmitter activity?
Appetite. 1988;11 Suppl 1:42-7.

Corsica JA, Spring BJ. Carbohydrate craving: a double-blind, placebo-controlled test of the self-medication hypothesis. *Eat Behav.* 2008 Dec;9(4):447-54. Epub 2008 Aug 4.

Sayegh R, Schiff I, Wurtman J, Spiers P, McDermott J, Wurtman R. The effect of a carbohydrate-rich beverage on mood, appetite, and cognitive function in women with premenstrual syndrome. *Obstet Gynecol.* 1995;86(4 Pt 1):520-8

Rapkin A. "The role of serotonin in premenstrual syndrome." *Clin Obstet Gyn* 1992;35(3):629-636

Lambert GW, Reid C, Kaye DM, Jennings GL, Esler MD. Effect of sunlight and season on serotonin turnover in the brain. *Lancet.* 2002 Dec 7;360(9348):1840-2.

Ferraro JS, Steger RW. Diurnal variations in brain serotonin are driven by the photic cycle and are not circadian in nature. *Brain Res.* 1990 Mar 26;512(1):121-4.

Wurtman R, Wurtman J, Regan M, McDermott J, Tsay R, Breu J. Effects of normal meals rich in carbohydrates or proteins on plasma tryptophan and tyrosine ratios. *Am J Clin Nutr.* 2003;77(1): 128-132.

Stephens NG, Parsons A, Schofield PM, Kelly F, Cheeseman K, Mitchinson MJ. Randomised controlled trial of vitamin E in patients with coronary disease: Cambridge Heart Antioxidant Study (CHAOS) *Lancet.* 1996;347(9004):781-6.

Cherubini A, Zuliani G, Costantini F, Pierdomenico SD, Volpato S, Mezzetti A, et al. VASA Study Group. High vitamin E plasma levels and low low-density lipoprotein oxidation are associated with the absence of atherosclerosis in octogenarians. *J Am Geriatr Soc.* 2001;49(5):651-4.

Gale CR, Ashurst HE, Powers HJ, Martyn CN. Antioxidant vitamin status and carotid atherosclerosis in the elderly. *Am J Clin Nutr.* 2001;74(3):402-8.

Riccioni G, D'Orazio N, Palumbo N, Bucciarelli V, Ilio E, Bazzano LA, et al. Relationship between plasma antioxidant concentrations and carotid intima-media thickness: the Asymptomatic Carotid Atherosclerotic Disease In Manfredonia Study. *Eur J Cardiovasc Prev Rehabil.* 2009;16(3):351-7.

Glynn RJ, Ridker PM, Goldhaber SZ, Zee RY, Buring JE. Effects of random allocation to vitamin E supplementation on the occurrence of venous thromboembolism: report from the Women's Health Study. *Circulation.* 2007;116(13):1497-503. Epub 2007 Sep 10.

Traber MG, Frei B, Beckman JS. Vitamin E revisited: do new data validate benefits for chronic disease prevention? *Curr Opin Lipidol.* 2008;19(1):30-8.

Wright ME, Lawson KA, Weinstein SJ, Pietinen P, Taylor PR, Virtamo J, et al. Higher baseline serum concentrations of vitamin E are associated with lower total and cause-specific mortality in the Alpha-Tocopherol, Beta-Carotene Cancer Prevention Study. *Am J Clin Nutr.* 2006;84(5):1200-7.

Meydani SN, Meydani M, Blumberg JB, Leka LS, Siber G, Loszewski R, et al. Vitamin E supplementation and in vivo immune response in healthy elderly subjects. A randomized controlled trial. *JAMA.* 1997;277(17):1380-6.

Kontush K, Schekatolina S. Vitamin E in neurodegenerative disorders: Alzheimer's disease.
Ann N Y Acad Sci. 2004;1031:249-62.

Sano M, Ernesto C, Thomas RG, Klauber MR, Schafer K, Grundman M, Woodbury P. A controlled trial of selegiline, alpha-tocopherol, or both as treatment for Alzheimer's disease. The Alzheimer's Disease Cooperative Study. *N Engl J Med.* 1997;336(17):1216-22.

ki KH, Losonczy KG, Izmirlian G, Foley DJ, Ross GW, Petrovitch H, et al. Association of vitamin E and C supplement use with cognitive function and dementia in elderly men. *Neurology.* 2000;54(6):1265-72.

Neuzil J, Weber T, Schröder A, Lu M, Ostermann G, Gellert N, et al. Induction of cancer cell apoptosis by alpha-tocopheryl succinate: molecular pathways and structural requirements. *FASEB J.* 2001;15(2):403-15.

Weber T, Lu M, Andera L, Lahm H, Gellert N, Fariss MW, et al. Vitamin E succinate is a potent novel antineoplastic agent with high selectivity and cooperativity with tumor necrosis factor-related apoptosis-inducing ligand (Apo2 ligand) in vivo. *Clin Cancer Res*. 2002;8(3):863-9.

Quin J, Engle D, Litwiller A, Peralta E, Grasch A, Boley T, et al. Vitamin E succinate decreases lung cancer tumor growth in mice. *J Surg Res*. 2005;127(2):139-43.

Guyton KZ, Kensler TW, Posner GH. Vitamin D and vitamin D analogs as cancer chemopreventive agents. *Nutr Rev*. 2003;61(7):227-38.

Welsh J, Wietzke JA, Zinser GM, Byrne B, Smith K, Narvaez CJ. Vitamin D-3 receptor as a target for breast cancer prevention. *J Nutr*. 2003;133(7 Suppl):2425S-2433S.

Holick MF. Vitamin D: importance in the prevention of cancers, Type 1 diabetes, heart disease, and osteoporosis. *Am J Clin Nutr*. 2004;79(3):362-71.

Zeitz U, Weber K, Soegiarto DW, Wolf E, Balling R, Erben RG. Impaired insulin secretory capacity in mice lacking a functional vitamin D receptor. *FASEB J*. 2003;17(3):509-11. Epub 2003 Jan 22.

Borissova AM, Tankova T, Kirilov G, Dakovska L, Kovacheva R. The effect of vitamin D3 on insulin secretion and peripheral insulin sensitivity in Type 2 diabetic patients. *Int J Clin Pract*. 2003;57(4):258-61.

Li YC, Kong J, Wei M, Chen ZF, Liu SQ, Cao LP. 1,25-Dihydroxyvitamin D(3) is a negative endocrine regulator of the renin-angiotensin system. *J Clin Invest*. 2002;110(2):229-38.

Vitamin D physiology. *Prog Biophys Mol Biol.* 2006;92(1):4-8. Epub 2006 Feb 28.

Plotnikoff GA, Quigley JM. Prevalence of severe hypovitaminosis D in patients with persistent, nonspecific musculoskeletal pain. *Mayo Clin Proc.* 2003;78(12):1463-70.

Broe KE, Chen TC, Weinberg J, Bischoff-Ferrari HA, Holick MF, Kiel DP. A higher dose of vitamin d reduces the risk of falls in nursing home residents: a randomized, multiple-dose study. *J Am Geriatr Soc.* 2007;55(2):234-9.

Feskanich D, Weber P, Willett WC, Rockett H, Booth SL, Colditz GA. Vitamin K intake and hip fractures in women: a prospective study. *Am J Clin Nutr.* 1999;69(1):74-9.

Garnero P, Hausherr E, Chapuy MC, Marcelli C, Grandjean H, Muller C, et al. Markers of bone resorption predict hip fracture in elderly women: the EPIDOS Prospective Study. *J Bone Miner Res.* 1996;11(10):1531-8.

Caraballo PJ, Heit JA, Atkinson EJ, Silverstein MD, O'Fallon WM, Castro MR, et al. 3rd
Long-term use of oral anticoagulants and the risk of fracture. *Arch Intern Med.* 1999 Aug 9-23;159(15):1750-6.

Kalkwarf HJ, Khoury JC, Bean J, Elliot JG. Vitamin K, bone turnover, and bone mass in girls. *Am J Clin Nutr.* 2004;80(4):1075-80.

Cockayne S, Adamson J, Lanham-New S, Shearer MJ, Gilbody S, Torgerson DJ. Vitamin K and the prevention of fractures: systematic review and meta-analysis of randomized controlled trials. *Arch Intern Med.* 2006;166(12):1256-61.

Braam LA, Knapen MH, Geusens P, Brouns F, Hamulyák K, Gerichhausen MJ, et al. Vitamin K1 supplementation retards bone loss in postmenopausal women between 50 and 60 years of age. *Calcif Tissue Int.* 2003 Jul;73(1):21-6.

Schurgers LJ, Dissel PE, Spronk HM, Soute BA, Dhore CR, Cleutjens JP, et al. Role of vitamin K and vitamin K-dependent proteins in vascular calcification. *Z Kardiol.* 2001;90 Suppl 3:57-63.

Jee-Aee Im, Byung-Pal Yu, Justin Y. Jeon, Sang-Hwan Kim. Relationship between osteocalcin and glucose metabolism in postmenopausal women. *Clinica Chimica Acta.* 2008; 396(1-2):66-69.

Lee NK, Sowa H, Hinoi E, Ferron M, Ahn JD, Confavreux C, et al. Endocrine regulation of energy metabolism by the skeleton. *Cell.* 2007; 130(3): 456–469.

Carbone LD, Barrow KD, Bush AJ, Boatright MD, Michelson JA, Pitts KA, et al. Effects of a low sodium diet on bone metabolism. *J Bone Miner Metab.* 2005;23(6):506-13.

Harris SS, Dawson-Hughes B. Caffeine and bone loss in healthy postmenopausal women.
Am J Clin Nutr. 1994;60(4):573-8.

Wallace K, Baron JA, Cole BF, Sandler RS, Karagas MR, Beach MA, et al. Effect of calcium supplementation on the risk of large bowel polyps. *J Natl Cancer Inst.* 2004;96(12):921-5.

Osganian SK, Stampfer MJ, Rimm E, Spiegelman D, Hu FB, Manson JE, et al. Vitamin C and risk of coronary heart disease in women. *J Am Coll Cardiol.* 2003;42(2):246-52.

Aggarwal BB, Bhardwaj A, Aggarwal RS, Seeram NP, Shishodia S, Takada Y. Role of resveratrol in prevention and therapy of cancer: preclinical and clinical studies. *Anticancer Res.* 2004 Sep-Oct;24(5A):2783-840.

Bradamante S, Barenghi L, Villa A. Cardiovascular protective effects of resveratrol. *Cardiovasc Drug Rev.* 2004 Fall;22(3):169-88.

Lu R, Serrero G. Resveratrol, a natural product derived from grape, exhibits antiestrogenic activity and inhibits the growth of human breast cancer cells. *J Cell Physiol.* 1999;179(3):297-304.

Bhat K, Lantvit D, Christov K, Mehta R. Estrogenic and Antiestrogenic Properties of Resveratrol in Mammary Tumor Models. *Cancer Res.* 2001; 61; 7456.

Li ZG, Hong T, Shimada Y, Komoto I, Kawabe A, Ding Y, et al. Suppression of *N*-nitrosomethylbenzylamine (NMBA)-induced esophageal tumorigenesis in F344 rats by resveratrol. *Carcinogenesis.* 2002; 23(9):1531-1536. doi: 10.1093/carcin/23.

Tessitore L, Davit A, Sarotto I, Caderni G. Resveratrol depresses the growth of colorectal aberrant crypt foci by affecting *bax* and *p21*[CIP] expression. *Carcinogenesis.* 2000; 21(8):1619-1622.

Boocock DJ, Faust GE, Patel KR, et al. Phase I dose escalation pharmacokinetic study in healthy volunteers of resveratrol, a potential cancer chemopreventive agent (*Cancer Epidemiol Biomarkers Prev.* 2007;16(6):1246-1252).

Ernster L, Dallner G. Biochemical, physiological and medical aspects of ubiquinone function (Biochim Biophys Acta. 1995;1271(1):195-204)

Wang GJ, Volkow ND, Fowler JS. The role of dopamine in motivation for food in humans: implications for obesity. *Expert Opin Ther Targets*. 2002;6(5):601-9.

Wang GJ, Volkow ND, Thanos PK, Fowler JS. Similarity between obesity and drug addiction as assessed by neurofunctional imaging: a concept review. *J Addict Dis.* 2004;23(3):39-53.

Brannan T, Martinez-Tica, J. Yahr. Effect of dietary protein on striatal dopamine formation following L-dopa administration: An in vivo study. *Neuropharmacology.* 1991: 30 (10):1125–1127.

Hood S, Cassidy P, Cossette Marie-Pierre, Weigl Y, Verwey M, Robinson B, et al. Endogenous Dopamine Regulates the Rhythm of Expression of the Clock Protein PER2 in the Rat Dorsal Striatum via Daily Activation of D2 Dopamine Receptors. *Journal of Neuroscience*, 2010; DOI: 10.1523/JNEUROSCI.2128-10.2010

Rabbani N, Alam SS, Riaz S, et al. High-dose thiamine therapy for patients with Type 2 diabetes and microalbuminuria: a randomized, double-blind placebo-controlled pilot study. Diabetologia. 2009;52:208-12.

Babaei-Jadidi R, Karachalias N, Ahmed N, et al. Prevention of incipient diabetic nephropathy by high-dose thiamine and benfotiamine. *Diabetes.* 2003;52:2110-20.

Koike H, Iijima M, Sugiura M, et al. Alcoholic neuropathy is clinicopathologically distinct from thiamine-deficiency neuropathy. *Ann Neurol* 2003;54:19-29.

Brown BG, Zhao XQ, Chalt A, et al. Simvastatin and niacin, antioxidant vitamins, or the combination for the prevention of coronary disease. *N Engl J Med.* 2001;345(22):1583-1592.

Cumming RG, Mitchell P, Smith W. Diet and cataract: the Blue Mountains Eye Study. *Ophthalmology.* 2000;107(3):450-456.

Elam M, Hunninghake DB, Davis KB, et al. Effects of niacin on lipid and lipoprotein levels and glycemic control in patients with diabetes and peripheral arterial disease: the ADMIT study: a randomized trial. Arterial Disease Multiple Intervention Trial. *JAMA.* 2000;284:1263-1270.

Jacques PF, Chylack LT Jr, Hankinson SE, et al. Long-term nutrient intake and early age related nuclear lens opacities. *Arch Ophthalmol.* 2001;119(7):1009-1019.

Torkos S. Drug-nutrient interactions: a focus on cholesterol-lowering agents. *Int J Integrative Med.* 2000;2(3):9-13.

Guyton JR. Niacin in cardiovascular prevention: mechanisms, efficacy, and safety. *Curr Opin Lipidol.* 2007;18(4):415-20.

Buvat DR. Use of metformin is a cause of vitamin B12 deficiency. *Am Fam Physician* 2004;69:264.

Den Elzen WP, Groeneveld Y, De Ruijter W, Souverijn JH, Le Cessie S, Assendelft WJ, et al. Long-term use of proton pump inhibitors (PPIs) and vitamin B12 status in elderly individuals. Aliment. *Pharmacol Ther* 2008;27:491-7.

Howden CW. Vitamin B12 levels during prolonged treatment with proton pump inhibitors. J *Clin Gastroenterol.* 2000;30:29-33.

Bottiglieri T. Folate, vitamin B12, and neuropsychiatric disorders. *Nutr Rev.* 1996;54:382-90.

The prevalence of vitamin B(12) deficiency in patients with Type 2 diabetes: a cross-sectional study. *J Am Board Fam Med.* 2009; 22(5):528-34.

Anesthesia paresthetica: nitrous oxide-induced cobalamin deficiency. *Neurology.* 1995; 45(8):1608-10.

Steiner I; Kidron D; Soffer D; Wirguin I; Abramsky O. Department of Neurology, Hadassah University Hospital, Jerusalem, Israel. Sensory peripheral neuropathy of vitamin B12 deficiency: a primary demyelinating disease? *J Neurol.* 1988; 235(3):163-4.
Plasma homocysteine levels and atherosclerosis in Japan: epidemiological study by use of carotid ultrasonography. *Stroke.* 2002; 33(9):2177-81.

Clarke R; Smith AD; Jobst KA; Refsum H; Sutton L; Ueland PM. Clinical Trial Service Unit, Nuffield Department of Clinical Medicine, Oxford, England. Folate, vitamin B12, and serum total homocysteine levels in confirmed Alzheimer disease. *Arch Neurol.* 1998; 55(11):1449-55.

Goodman BP; Chong BW; Patel AC; Fletcher GP; Smith BE Department of Neurology, Mayo Clinic Scottsdale, Scottsdale, AZ. Copper deficiency myeloneuropathy resembling B12 deficiency: partial resolution of MR imaging findings with copper supplementation. *AJNR Am J Neuroradiol.* 2006; 27(10):2112-4.

Food and Nutrition Board, Institute of Medicine. Iron. Dietary reference intakes for vitamin A, vitamin K, boron, chromium, copper, iodine, iron, manganese, molybdenum, nickel, silicon, vanadium, and zinc. Washington D.C.: National Academy Press; 2001:290-393. (National Academy Press).

Thomas DG, Grant SL, Aubuchon-Endsley NL. The role of iron in neurocognitive development. *Dev Neuropsychol.* 2009;34(2):196-222.

Earley CJ, Connor JR, Beard JL, Malecki EA, Epstein DK, Allen RP. Abnormalities in CSF concentrations of ferritin and transferrin in restless legs syndrome. *Neurology.* 2000;54(8):1698-1700.

Kagan BL; Sultzer DL; Rosenlicht N; Gerner RH. Department of Psychiatry, West Los Angeles VA Medical Center, CA. Oral S-adenosylmethionine in depression: a randomized, double-blind, placebo-controlled trial. *Am J Psychiatry.* 1990; 147(5):591-5)

De Jager J, Kooy A, Lehert P, Wulffelé MG, van der Kolk J, Bets D, et al. Long term treatment with metformin in patients with Type 2 diabetes and risk of vitamin B-12 deficiency: randomised placebo controlled trial. *BMJ.* 2010;340:c2181.
van der Mooren MJ; Wouters MG; Blom HJ; Schellekens LA; Eskes TK; Rolland R. Department of Obstetrics & Gynecology, University Hospital Nijmegen Sint Radboud, The Netherlands. Hormone replacement therapy may reduce high serum homocysteine in postmenopausal women. *Eur J Clin Invest.* 1994; 24(11):733-6.

Devine A, Criddle RA, Dick IM, Kerr DA, Prince RL. Department of Medicine, University of Western Australia, Sir Charles Gairdner Hospital, Nedlands. A longitudinal study of the effect of sodium and calcium intakes on regional bone density in postmenopausal women. *Am J Clin Nutr.* 1995;62(4):740-5.

Neuropeptide Y acts directly in the periphery on fat tissue and mediates stress-induced obesity and metabolic syndrome. *Nature Medicine* 13, 803 - 811 (2007). Published online: 1 July 2007 | Corrected online: 24 July 2007 | doi:10.1038/nm1611.

Deborah A. Siwik, Patrick J. Pagano, and Wilson S. Colucci. Oxidative stress regulates collagen synthesis and matrix metalloproteinase activity in cardiac fibroblasts. *Am J Physiol Cell Physiol* January 1, 2001 vol. 280 no. 1 C53-C60.

Hyejin Lee, Christopher M. Overall, Christopher A. McCulloch, and Jaro Sodek A Critical Role for the Membrane-type 1 Matrix Metalloproteinase in Collagen. *Phagocytosis Mol Biol Cell.* 2006 November; 17(11): 4812–4826.

Geesin JC, Gordon JS, Berg RA. Regulation of collagen synthesis in human dermal fibroblasts by the sodium and magnesium salts of ascorbyl-2-phosphate. *Skin Pharmacol.* 1993;6(1):65-71.

Hata R, Senoo H. L-ascorbic acid 2-phosphate stimulates collagen accumulation, cell proliferation, and formation of a three-dimensional tissuelike substance by skin fibroblasts. *J Cell Physiol.* 1989;138(1):8-16.

Tajima S, Pinnell SR. Ascorbic acid preferentially enhances type I and III collagen gene transcription in human skin fibroblasts. *J Dermatol Sci.* 1996;11(3):250-3.

Nusgens BV, Humbert P, Rougier A, et al. Topically applied vitamin C enhances the mRNA level of collagens I and III, their processing enzymes and tissue inhibitor of matrix metalloproteinase 1 in the human dermis. *J Invest Dermatol.* 2001;116(6):853-9.

T. Mitsuishi, T. Shimoda, Y. Mitsui, Y. Kuriyana, S. Kawana. The effects of topical application of phytonadione, retinol and vitamins C and E on infraorbital dark circles and wrinkles of the lower eyelids. *Journal of Cosmetic Dermatology.* 2004; 3;73-75.

Draelos Z, Jacobson E, Kim H, Kim M, Jacobson M. Department of Dermatology, Wake Forest University School of Medicine, NC, Department of Pharmacology and Toxicology, University of Arizona, AZ, Arizona Cancer Center, University of Arizona. A pilot study evaluating the efficacy of topically applied niacin derivatives for treatment of female pattern alopecia.

Bissett DL, Oblong JE, Berge CA. Niacinamide: A B vitamin that improves aging facial skin appearance. *Dermatol Surg.* 2005;31(7 Pt 2):860-5; discussion 865.

Bissett DL, Miyamoto K, Sun P, Li J, Berge CA. Topical niacinamide reduces yellowing, wrinkling, red blotchiness, and hyperpigmented spots in aging facial skin. *Int J Cosmet Sci.* 2004;26(5):231-8.

Kawada A, Konishi N, Oiso N, Kawara S, Date A. Evaluation of anti-wrinkle effects of a novel cosmetic containing niacinamide. *J Dermatol.* 2008;35(10):637-42.

Fu JJ, Hillebrand GG, Raleigh P, Li J, Marmor MJ, Bertucci V, et al. A randomized, controlled comparative study of the wrinkle reduction benefits of a cosmetic niacinamide/peptide/retinyl propionate product regimen vs. a prescription 0.02% tretinoin product regimen. *Br J Dermatol.* 2010;162(3):647-54.

Christman JC, Fix DK, Lucus SC, Watson D, Desmier E, Wilkerson RJ, et al. Two randomized, controlled, comparative studies of the stratum corneum integrity benefits of two cosmetic niacinamide/glycerin body moisturizers vs. conventional body moisturizers. *J Drugs Dermatol.* 2012;11(1):22-9.

Draelos ZD, Ertel K, Berge C. Niacinamide-containing facial moisturizer improves skin barrier and benefits subjects with rosacea. *Cutis.* 2005;76(2):135-41.

May JM, Qu ZC, Mendiratta S. Protection and recycling of alpha-tocopherol in human erythrocytes by intracellular ascorbic acid. *Arch Biochem Biophys.* 1998;349(2):281-9.

Klock J, Ikeno H, Ohmori K, et al. Sodium ascorbyl phosphate shows in vitro and in vivo efficacy in the prevention and treatment of acne vulgaris. *Int J Cosmet Sci.* 2005;27(3):171-6.

Kameyama K, Sakai C, Kondoh S, et al. Inhibitory effect of magnesium L-ascorbyl-2-phosphate (VC-PMG) on melanogenesis in vitro and in vivo. *J Am Acad Dermatol.* 1996;34(1):29-33.

Katiyar SK. Skin photoprotection by green tea: antioxidant and immunomodulatory effects. *Curr Drug Targets Immune Endocr Metabol Disord.* 2003;3(3):234-42.

Traikovich SS. Use of topical ascorbic acid and its effects on photodamaged skin topography. *Arch Otolaryngol Head Neck Surg.* 1999;125(10):1091-8.

Myllyla R, Majamaa K, Gunzler V, Hanauske-Abel HM, Kivirikko KI. Ascorbate is consumed stoichiometrically in the uncoupled reactions catalyzed by prolyl 4-hydroxylase and lysyl hydroxylase. *J Biol Chem.* 1984;259(9):5403-5.

Humbert PG, Haftek M, Creidi P, et al. Topical ascorbic acid on photoaged skin. Clinical, topographical and ultrastructural evaluation: double-blind study vs. placebo. *Exp Dermatol.* 2003;12(3):237-44.

Fitzpatrick RE, Rostan EF. Double-blind, half-face study comparing topical vitamin C and vehicle for rejuvenation of photodamage. *Dermatol Surg.* 2002;28(3):231-6.

Farris PK. Topical vitamin C: a useful agent for treating photoaging and other dermatologic conditions. *Dermatol Surg.* 2005;31(7 Pt 2):814-7.

Varani J, Warner RL, Gharaee-Kermani M et al. Vitamin A antagonizes decreased cell growth and elevated collagen-degrading matrix metalloproteinases and stimulates collagen accumulation in naturally aged human skin. *J Invest Dermatol.* 2000; 114:480–6.

Griffiths C, Russman A, Majmudar G, Singer R, Hamilton T, Voorhees J. Restoration of Collagen Formation in Photodamaged Human Skin by Tretinoin (Retinoic Acid) *N Engl J Med.* 1993; 329:530-535

Bulengo-Ransby SM, Griffiths CE, Kimbrough-Green CK, Finkel LJ, Hamilton TA, Ellis CN, et al. Department of Dermatology, University of Michigan Medical Center, Ann Arbor: Topical tretinoin (retinoic acid) therapy for hyperpigmented lesions caused by inflammation of the skin in black patients. *N Engl J Med.* 1993;328(20):1438-43.

Rafal ES, Griffiths CE, Ditre CM, Finkel LJ, Hamilton TA, Ellis CN, et al. Department of Dermatology, University of Michigan Medical Center, Ann Arbor Topical tretinoin (retinoic acid) treatment for liver spots associated with photodamage. *N Engl J Med.* 1992;326(6):368-74.

Griffiths CE, Finkel LJ, Ditre CM, Hamilton TA, Ellis CN, Voorhees JJ. Department of Dermatology, University of Michigan Medical Center, Ann Arbor. Topical tretinoin (retinoic acid) improves melasma. A vehicle-controlled, clinical trial. *Br J Dermatol.* 1993;129(4):415-21

Robinson LR, Fitzgerald NC, Doughty DG, Dawes NC, Berge CA, Bissett DL. Topical palmitoyl pentapeptide provides improvement in photoaged human facial skin. *Int J Cosmet Sci.* 2005;27(3):155-60.

Blanes-Mira C, Clemente J, Jodas G, Gil A, Fernández-Ballester G, Ponsati B, Gutierrez L, Pérez-Payá E, Ferrer-Montiel A. A synthetic hexapeptide (Argireline) with antiwrinkle activity. *Int J Cosmet Sci.* 2002;24(5):303-10.

Brown RG, Button GM, Smith JT. Changes in collagen metabolism caused by feeding diets low in inorganic sulfur. *J Nutr.* 1965;87(2):228-32.

Marini H, Polito F, Altavilla D, Irrera N, Minutoli L, Calò M, et al. Genistein aglycone improves skin repair in an incisional model of wound healing: a comparison with raloxifene and oestradiol in ovariectomized rats. *Br J Pharmacol.* 2010;160(5):1185-94.

Polito F, Marini H, Bitto A, Irrera N, Vaccaro M, Adamo EB, et al. Genistein aglycone, a soy-derived isoflavone, improves skin changes induced by ovariectomy in rats. *Br J Pharmacol.* 2012;165(4):994-1005.

Kang S, Chung JH, Lee JH, Fisher G, Wan YS, Duell E, Voorhees J. Topical N-Acetyl Cysteine and Genistein Prevent Ultraviolet-Light-Induced Signaling That Leads to Photoaging in Human Skin in vivo. *Journal of Investigative Dermatology.* 2003;120, 835–841.

Khanna S, Venojarvi M, Roy S, Sharma N, Trikha P, Bagchi D, et al. Dermal wound healing properties of redox-active grape seed Proanthocyanidins. *Free Radical Biology and Medicine.* 2002; 33 (8):1089–10.

Stahl W, Sies H. Carotenoids and Protection against Solar UV Radiation. *Skin Pharmacol Appl Skin Physiol.* 2002;15:291-296.

Valacchi G, Pecorelli A, Mencarelli M, Maioli E, Davis PA. Beta-carotene prevents ozone-induced proinflammatory markers in murine skin. *Toxicol Ind Health.* 2009 May-Jun;25(4-5):241-7.

Ribaya-Mercado JD, Garmyn M, Gilchrest BA, Russell RM. Skin lycopene is destroyed preferentially over beta-carotene during ultraviolet irradiation in humans. *J Nutr.* 1995;125(7):1854-9.

Bagchi D, Sen C, Ray S, Das D, Bagchi M, Preuss H, et al. Molecular mechanisms of cardioprotection by a novel grape seed proanthocyanidin extract. *Mutation Research/Fundamental and Molecular Mechanisms of Mutagenesis*, volumes 523–524, February–March 2003, Pages 87–97.

Vitseva O, Varghese S, Chakrabarti S, Folts JD, Freedman JE. Grape seed and skin extracts inhibit platelet function and release of reactive oxygen intermediates. *J Cardiovasc Pharmacol.* 2005; 46 (4): 445–51.

Inflamm-Aging, Cytokines and Aging: State of the Art, New Hypotheses on the Role of Mitochondria and New Perspectives from Systems Biology. *Curr Pharm Des.* 2006;12(24):3161-71.

Influence of Gastric Acidity on Bacterial and Parasitic Enteric Infections *A Perspective Annals internal medicine.* February 1, 1973 vol. 78 no. 2 271-276.

Ruddell WSJ, Axon ATR, Findlay JM, Bartholomew BA, Hill MJ. The effect of cimetidine on the gastric bacterial microflora. *Lancet* 1980; i:672-674.

Ruddell WSJ, Losowsky MS. Severe diarrhea due to small intestinal colonisation during cimetidine treatment. *Br Med J.* 1980;3:273.

Sharma BK, Santana IA, Wood EC, Walt RP, Pereira M, Noone P, et al. Intragastric bacterial activity and nitrosation before, during, and after treatment with omeprazole. *Br Med J.* 1984;289:717-719.

Linsky, A, Gupta K, Lawler E, Fonda J, Hermos J. Proton Pump Inhibitors and Risk for Recurrent Clostridium difficile Infection . *Arch Intern Med.* 2010;170(9):772-778.

Influence of Gastric Acidity on Bacterial and Parasitic Enteric Infections

A Perspective. *Annals Internal Medicine*. February 1, 1973 vol. 78 no. 2 271-276.

Fried M, Siegrist H, Frei R, Froehlich F, Duroux P, Thorens J, et al. Duodenal bacterial overgrowth during treatment in outpatients with omeprazole. *Gut.* 1994;35(1):23-6.

Patel TA, Abraham P, Ashar VJ, Bhatia SJ, Anklesaria PS. Gastric bacterial overgrowth accompanies profound acid suppression. *Indian J Gastroenterol.* 1995;14(4):134-6.

Wang K, Lin HJ, Perng CL, Tseng GY, Yu KW, Chang FY, et al. The effect of H2-receptor antagonist and proton pump inhibitor on microbial proliferation in the stomach. *Hepatogastroenterology.* 2004 Sep-Oct;51(59):1540-3.

R. Hughes, E.A.M. Magee and S. Bingham. Protein Degradation in the Large Intestine: Relevance to Colorectal Cancer *Curr. Issues Intest. Microbiol.* 2000. 1(2): 51-58.

Levy, R, Brouns F, Beckers E. Is the gut an athletic organ? Digestion, absorption and exercise. *Clinical Gastroenterology and Hepatology,* 2005.

Inflammatory networks in ageing, age-related diseases and longevity. *Mech Ageing Dev.* 2007;128(1):83-91. Epub 2006 Nov 21.

Low grade inflammation and coronary heart disease: prospective study and updated meta-analyses. *BMJ.* 2000; 321(7255): 199–204.

Chronic inflammation and the effect of IGF-I on muscle strength and power in older persons. *AJP Endo.* 2003;284(3):E481-E487.

Normal-weight obese syndrome: early inflammation? *American Journal of Clinical Nutrition.* 2007: 85(1):40-45.

Normal weight obesity: a risk factor for cardiometabolic dysregulation and cardiovascular mortality. *Eur Heart J.* 2010; 31(6): 737-746.

Effects of transdermal testosterone on bone and muscle in older men with low bioavailable testosterone levels. *J Gerontol A Biol Sci Med Sci.* 2001;56(5):M266-72.

Testosterone but not estradiol level is positively related to muscle strength and physical performance independent of muscle mass: a cross-sectional study in 1489 older men. *Eur J Endocrinol.* 2011;164(5):811-7. Epub 2011 Feb 23.

Bioavailable Testosterone and Depressed Mood in Older Men: The Rancho Bernardo Study. *The Journal of Clinical Endocrinology & Metabolism.* 1999; 84(2):573-577.

Deficiencies in circulating testosterone and dehydroepiandrosterone sulphate, and depression in men with systolic chronic heart failure. *Eur J Heart Fail.* 2010;12 (9): 966-973.

Low free testosterone is associated with heart failure mortality in older men referred for coronary angiography. *Eur J Heart Fail.* 2011;13(5): 482-488.

Testosterone Deficiency As a Risk Factor for Hip. *American Journal of the Medical Sciences.* 1992; 304(1).

The Effects of Serum Testosterone, Estradiol, and Sex Hormone Binding Globulin Levels on Fracture Risk in Older Men. *The Journal of Clinical Endocrinology & Metabolism.* 2009; 94(9): 3337-3346.

Bremner W, Vitiello M, Prinz P. Loss of Circadian Rhythmicity in Blood Testosterone Levels with Aging in Normal Men *The Journal of Clinical Endocrinology & Metabolism.* 1983; 56(6): 1278-1281.

Amore M, et al. Partial androgen deficiency, depression and testosterone treatment in aging men. *Aging Clinical and Experimental Research.* 2009;21:1.

Emmelot-Vonk MH, et al. Effect of testosterone supplementation on functional mobility, cognition, and other parameters in older men: A randomized controlled trial. *JAMA.* 2008;299:39.

Barrett-Connor E, von Mühlen D, Kritz-Silverstein D. Bioavailable Testosterone and Depressed Mood in Older Men: The Rancho Bernardo Study. *Endocrinology & Metabolism.* 1999; 84(2): 573-577.

Sattler F, Castaneda-Sceppa C, Binder E, Schroeder ET, Wang Y, Bhasin S, et al. Testosterone and Growth Hormone Improve Body Composition and Muscle Performance in Older Men. *The Journal of Clinical Endocrinology & Metabolism.* 2009; 94(6):1991-2001.

Rariy C, Ratcliffe S, Weinstein R, Bhasin S, Blackman M, Cauley J, et al. Higher Serum Free Testosterone Concentration in Older Women Is Associated with Greater Bone Mineral Density, Lean Body Mass, and Total Fat Mass: The Cardiovascular Health Study. *The Journal of Clinical Endocrinology & Metabolism.* 2011; 96(4):989-996.

Hofling M, Hirschberg AL, Skoog L, Tani E, Hägerström T, von Schoultz B. Testosterone inhibits estrogen/progestogen-induced breast cell proliferation in postmenopausal women. *Menopause*. 2007 Mar-Apr;14(2):183-90.

Barqawi E D. Crawford Testosterone Replacement Therapy and the Risk of Prostate Cancer. Is there a link? *International J Impotence Research*. 2006;18(4):323-328.

Stress and premature menopause. *C R Acad Sci III.* 1995;318(6):691-8.

Changes in the Serum Cholesterol and Blood Clotting Time in Men Subjected to Cyclic Variation of Occupational Stress. *Circulation.* 1958;17:852-861.

Chandola T. et al. Work Stress and Coronary Heart Disease: What are the mechanisms? *European Heart Journal*, January 2008.

Soares CN, Joffe H, Steiner M. Menopause and mood. *Clin Obstet Gynecol*. 2004;47(3):576-91.

Cohen LS, Soares CN, Vitonis AF, Otto MW, Harlow BL. Risk for new onset of depression during the menopausal transition: the Harvard study of moods and cycles. *Arch Gen Psychiatry*. 2006;63(4):385-90.

Pilkington P, Windsor T, Crisp D. Volunteering and Subjective Well-Being in Midlife and Older Adults: The Role of Supportive Social Networks. *J Gerontol B Psychol Sci Soc Sci.* 2012.

Piliavin JA, Siegl E. Health Benefits of Volunteering in the Wisconsin Longitudinal Study. *Journal of Health and Social Behavior*. 2007;48(4):450-464.

Cohen LS, Soares CN, Vitonis AF, Otto MW, Harlow BL. Risk for new onset of depression during the menopausal transition: the Harvard study of moods and cycles. *Arch Gen Psychiatry*. 2006;63(4):385-90.

Murphy PJ, Cambell SS. Sex hormones, sleep, and core body temperature in older postmenopausal women. *Sleep*. 2007;30 (12):1788-94.

Tom SE, Kuh D, Guralnik JM, Mishra GD. Self-reported sleep difficulty during the menopausal transition: results from a prospective cohort study. *Menopause*. Nov-Dec 2010;17(6):1128-35.

Claudia P, Andrea C, Chiara C, Stefano L, Giuseppe M, Vincenzo DL. Panic disorder in menopause: a case control study. *Maturitas*. 2004;48(2):147-54.

Estrogen and skin. An overview. *Am J Clin Dermatol*. 2001;2(3):143-50.

Serotonin Receptor Modulation by Estrogen in Discrete Brain Nuclei. *Neuroendocrinology*. 1982;35:287-291 (DOI: 10.1159/000123396).

Estrogen control of central neurotransmission: effect on mood, mental state, and memory. *Cell Mol Neurobiol*. 1996;16(3):325-44.

Stimulatory effects of estrogen and progesterone on proliferation and differentiation of normal human osteoblast-like cells in vitro. *Biochemical and Biophysical Research Communications*. 1992; 186(1):54-60.

Progesterone induces changes in sleep comparable to those of agonistic GABAA receptor modulators. *AJP – Endo.* 1996;271(4):E763-E772.

Allopregnanolone Affects Sleep in a Benzodiazepine-Like Fashion. *J. Pharmacol. Exp. Ther.* 1997;282:(3):1213-1218.

Increased Progesterone Production During the Luteal Phase of Menstruation May Decrease Anesthetic Requirement. *Anethesia & Analgesia.* 2005;101(4):1007-1011.

Progesterone decreases sevoflurane requirement in male mice: a dose–response study. *Br. J. Anaesth.* 2010;104 (5): 603-605.

Hak AE, Pols H, Visser T, Drexhage H, Hofman A, Witteman, J. Subclinical Hypothyroidism Is an Independent Risk Factor for Atherosclerosis and Myocardial Infarction in Elderly Women: The Rotterdam Study. *Annals of Internal Medicine.* 2000; 132(4).

About Dr Eudene Harry

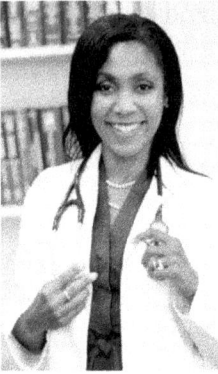

We only have one body, one mind, and one lifetime to make the best of it. I believe that the body behaves as a complete, integrative system, and without this optimal balance we are not living to our fullest potential. All the years I heard my grandmother say "one ounce of prevention is better than a pound of cure", I thought "oh boy" another quirky saying. Now, the older I get I am seeing and living the wisdom and value of her words.

Being an Emergency Room Physician for well over 12 years and working in some of the largest and busiest ER's in the State, I treated my share of patients with many issues. Some patients I am proud to say were saved, cured, and helped to find a remedy to their specific illness. Then there were many times where I wished there was more I could have done. I became frustrated with time after time knowing there must be more treatments available that may complement or enhance traditional western medicine to optimize health. My oath and responsibility as a Medical Doctor is to treat my patients to the best of my ability and I believe that Integrative Medicine is the best way to do so

Integrative Holistic Medicine combines the best of conventional medicine and evidence based complementary medicine to achieve a natural balance that enables the healing process. This means supplying the body what it needs to achieve balance can only augment and accelerate any healing process. This does not in any way replace or reject "mainstream medicine" but rather takes a complete body system approach to health. This form of medicine acknowledges the science of the mind, body connection, views the relationship between physician and patient as a partnership and an important part of the healing process. Finally, the focus is on optimizing health and not the absence of disease.

This understanding is why I have been successful in marrying Traditional and Holistic Medicine in my practice and in daily living.

Throughout my career I have and plan to continue bringing the message of complete health and balance to my patients as well as the community. I have been a guest speaker at local colleges and school programs to involve our youth in ending childhood obesity and promoting nutrition for brain power. I have written for several publications including Orlando Medical News, Ladies Home Journal, Self.com and the Southwest Bulletin. As an educator I have participated in "Ask the Doctor" radio programs and spoken at multiple seminars designed to educate the general public and health care professionals alike. I feel so fortunate to be able to provide valuable information to my patients as well as the community. With this book I hope to provide the tools and strategies that will allow all of us to take responsibility and achieve the ultimate well-being.

The juggling act of everyday life is difficult, this will never change. As a mother of two children, a wife and a Physician truly dedicated to her patients I understand the complexity of daily life. So often we have the "I can handle it all" mentality. This in no way creates balance. We all need to take a step (or two) back, evaluate what are necessities vs. desires, find a dependable support system, make a realistic plan, and feed our mind, body, and spirit. This will restore the vitality and vigor we all have inside. I hope this book helps ignite the flame within and get you on your way to living healthy, looking younger, and achieving optimal health.

Dr. Eudene Harry

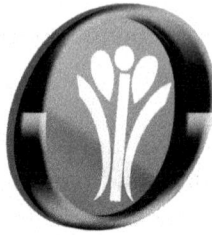

Oasis Wellness and Rejuvenation Center

Dr. Eudene Harry

4125 Hunters Park Suite 117
Orlando, Florida 32837

407-354-0500

rejuvenateandrestore@gmail.com

drharry@livinghealthylookingyounger.com

Visit us on the web at:

www. LivingHealthyLookingYounger.com

www.ingramcontent.com/pod-product-compliance
Lightning Source LLC
Chambersburg PA
CBHW070519200326
41519CB00013B/2851